Incredible
Orgasms

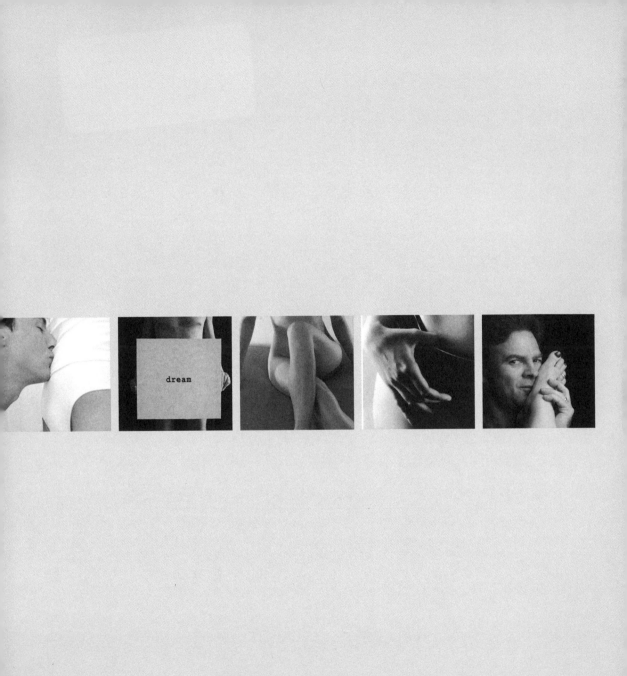

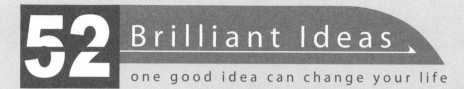

52 Brilliant Ideas

one good idea can change your life

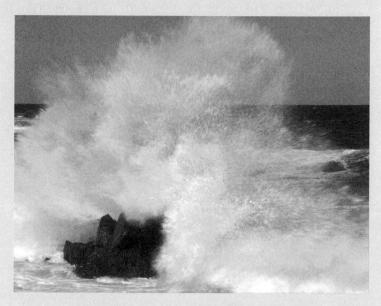

Incredible Orgasms

yes, yes, Yes, YES, YESSS!

Marcelle Perks

A Perigee Book

A PERIGEE BOOK
Published by the Penguin Group
Penguin Group (USA) Inc.
375 Hudson Street, New York, New York 10014, USA
Penguin Group (Canada), 90 Eglinton Avenue East, Suite 700, Toronto, Ontario M4P 2Y3, Canada
(a division of Pearson Penguin Canada Inc.)
Penguin Books Ltd., 80 Strand, London WC2R 0RL, England
Penguin Group Ireland, 25 St. Stephen's Green, Dublin 2, Ireland (a division of Penguin Books Ltd.)
Penguin Group (Australia), 250 Camberwell Road, Camberwell, Victoria 3124, Australia (a division of Pearson Australia Group Pty. Ltd.)
Penguin Books India Pvt. Ltd., 11 Community Centre, Panchsheel Park, New Delhi—110 017, India
Penguin Group (NZ), Cnr. Airborne and Rosedale Roads, Albany, Auckland 1310, New Zealand (a division of Pearson New Zealand Ltd.)
Penguin Books (South Africa) (Pty.) Ltd., 24 Sturdee Avenue, Rosebank, Johannesburg 2196, South Africa

Penguin Books Ltd., Registered Offices: 80 Strand, London WC2R 0RL, England

While the author has made every effort to provide accurate telephone numbers and Internet addresses at the time of publication, neither the publisher nor the author assumes any responsibility for errors, or for changes that occur after publication. Further, the publisher does not have any control over and does not assume any responsibility for author or third-party websites or their content.

First American edition: January 2007
Originally published in Great Britain in 2006 by The Infinite Ideas Company Limited.

Library of Congress Cataloging-in-Publication Data

Perks, Marcelle.
    Incredible orgasms : yes, yes, Yes, Yes, YESSS! / Marcelle Perks.
        p.   cm. — (52 brilliant ideas)
    "A Perigee book."
    Includes index.
    ISBN: 978-0-399-53303-7 (trade pbk.)
        1. Sex instruction.   2. Orgasm.   I. Title.

    HQ31.P449 2007
    613.9'6—dc22

                                        2006050669

PRINTED IN THE UNITED STATES OF AMERICA

10 9 8 7 6 5 4 3 2 1

PUBLISHER'S NOTE: Neither the publisher nor the author is engaged in rendering professional advice or services to the individual reader. The ideas, procedures, and suggestions contained in this book are not intended as a substitute for consulting with your physician. All matters regarding your health require medical supervision. Neither the author nor the publisher shall be liable or responsible for any loss or damage allegedly arising from any information or suggestion in this book.

Most Perigee Books are available at special quantity discounts for bulk purchases for sales promotions, premiums, fund-raising, or educational use. Special books, or book excerpts, can also be created to fit specific needs. For details, write: Special Markets, The Berkley Publishing Group, 375 Hudson Street, New York, New York 10014.

Brilliant ideas

Brilliant features

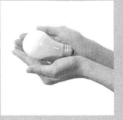

Each chapter of this book is designed to provide you with an inspirational idea that you can read quickly and put into practice right away.

Throughout you'll find four features that will help you get to the heart of the idea:

- *Here's an idea for you* Take it on board and give it a try—right here, right now. Get an idea of how well you're doing so far.

- *Try another idea* If this idea looks like a life-changer then there's no time to lose. *Try another idea* will point you straight to a related tip to enhance and expand on the first.

- *Defining ideas* Words of wisdom from masters and mistresses of the art, plus some interesting hangers-on.

- *How did it go?* If at first you do succeed, try to hide your amazement. If, on the other hand, you don't, then this is where you'll find a Q and A that highlights common problems and how to get over them.

Introduction

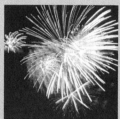

You're probably thinking that the kind of person who writes about sex must be some kind of sexpert or, at the very least, an enthusiastic sexpot. Actually when I was commissioned to write this book I was just recovering from a miscarriage. It's true that I write about sex as an erotic writer and in nonfiction pieces where I get to ask doctors thousands of questions. But the main trick to having good orgasms, like writing a book, is to have lots of enthusiasm and a healthy dose of curiosity. It's been a great experience tracking down medical stuff, reading lots of books, calling all kinds of people, and surfing loads of X-rated websites.

There's no specific audience for this book. You have to be female because it's aimed at women, but there's something for everyone whether you're still a virgin or an experienced seductress who likes to paint the town red on a Saturday night. Perhaps you're young, or maybe you're already a great-grandmother; some of you might have to work around your physical disabilities, others will have mental blocks that make their lives difficult. Whatever point we start off from, all of us have our positive points and "shadow" sides to wrestle with.

The information is broadly aimed at heterosexuals, although I hope that lesbian and transgendered women will find their interests well served, too. In the text you'll notice that when I get tired of using the word "partner" I've used the personal pronouns he/his/him to refer to your other half; this is simply for convenience and due to word space limitations. I started off going for his/her, but it just got too clumsy. Apologies in advance for readers with female partners; no presumption is intended. Similarly, if you're single or don't have a regular partner, please don't cringe at all the tips aimed at regular couples. Just store the advice up for the future, for a time when you can test the ideas out.

My main aim is to help you improve your sex life, and although I can't guarantee you'll have an orgasm (about 10 percent of women say they *never* climax) there are lots of ideas here that will at least put some fun and interest back into the mix. There are plenty of practical tips and tricks for better techniques to help you along, but they're accompanied by parts devoted to improving your mental outlook. Good sex really is a mixture of biology and psychology. I also make the connection between sex and having babies, something most sex books leave out—as if the two had nothing to do with each other! There's a bit of delving into history, philosophy, sexual politics, and anthropology. A lot of ideas here are bunched together for the first time, which means there's plenty to think about.

Where possible I've included the latest scientific research, although once you get the "hot favorites" like the G-spot and multiple orgasms out of the way, there's surprisingly little information out there on topics that you'd think would be well researched. On occasions where there's been no information I've borrowed ideas from other disciplines like sports science, or made up ideas on the spot (as in idea 23, *Sex in water*).

Don't feel that you have to try out all the suggestions. Some may not be appropriate for you and I haven't road-tested each and every one myself. Not all of the issues presented are light and fluffy, and I haven't shied away from uncomfortable ones like domestic abuse and vulvar discomfort. There's an honest attempt to present the real deal, warts and all, rather than saccharine secrets for Stepford Wives.

My best advice is to focus on changing your attitudes toward sex. Good sex is not the exclusive plaything of supermodels and Oscar-winning actresses (you'll be shocked when you read idea 47, *Hedonism*). Women like Jane Juska, who wrote an autobiographical account—*A Round-heeled Woman*—of her attempts to date men in her sixties through a personal ad, show us that our desires remain vibrant for our whole life. Likewise, those who are ill also strive for pleasure. Lucy Grealy, who underwent years of surgery on her facial bone cancer, gives a painstakingly honest account of her search for love in *Autobiography of a Face*. Journalist Kath Duncan, who also happens to be a congenital amputee with one arm and one leg, made the film *My One-legged Dream Lover* (1999) about her encounters with amputee lovers who fetishize her body. These personal revelations on sensitive areas, previously considered taboo, help us to become more embracing and accepting of our own and each other's sexualities.

What we've got in common is that we're all looking for "it." I hope this book helps you to discover the sizzling side to your sexuality and that the neighbors start complaining about your blissful screams!

"On me your voice falls as they say love should, Like an enormous yes."
PHILIP LARKIN, *For Sidney Bechet*—probably the best love poem in the English language, although actually he's talking about jazz...

Defining idea...

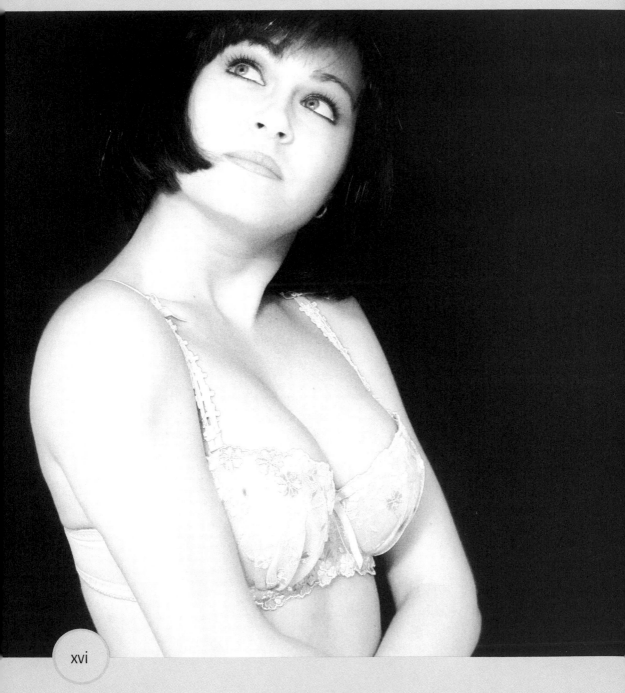

1

What sexual thoughts are you made of?

Before we even think physical, we need to probe the most important part—what's on your mind.

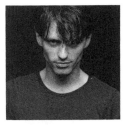

The good news is that sex is universal and democratic, and can be enjoyed whether you're young or old, able-bodied or not, thin or fat, plain or pretty.

In theory, expressing our sexuality has never been easier. Women now have more opportunities and freedom, a range of contraceptive options, speed dating, online chat sites, and amazing sex aids. You'd think we've never had it so good, and yet, according to the Durex 2004 Global Sex Survey, only 35 percent of women climax every time they have sex. Studies show around 40 percent of women suffer from sexual dysfunction and about a fifth of us have low levels of libido. Around 10 percent of women claim they never have orgasms. That means most of us have room for improvement.

Of course, achieving a climax is not everything, and you can have good sex without the physical "release" of an orgasm. Sometimes our expectations are simply too

Here's an idea for you... **Imagine you are your partner telling someone else about what you're like in bed. Highlight your good points, and list any features that are particularly sexy. See how many positive things you can relate about yourself. Often we exaggerate, but the little white lies could later become reality!**

high. When researchers Hartman and Fithian wired up twenty women in a laboratory study who reckoned they couldn't climax, 75 percent of them underwent the physical responses of orgasm without even realizing it. They *imagined* it would be better than it was! Although we can say, medically, that an orgasm is a reflex of the PC (pubococcygeus) muscles when they spasm rhythmically at 0.8 second intervals, it's still hard for us to describe what an orgasm actually feels like. Men have the physical reality of their ejaculation, but the female orgasm is more complex and mysterious. We have more orgasm possibilities (clitoral, G-spot, vaginal, full body, U- and X-spots), and so we can't compare our orgasms to that scene in *When Harry Met Sally*. Even our orgasm responses aren't neutral. Sex researchers say we each have an "orgasm fingerprint" that affects how we react to orgasm. Some of us scream because we think that's just how we should respond!

Don't worry, then, about how you should feel or act; concentrate on your mental approach to sexual pleasure. We expect sex to be wild and instinctive but we don't come to sex neutrally; it's an emotional minefield that's affected by our upbringing and experience. To improve things, think positive. If you anticipate that it will be a good experience, regardless of the actual performance, you're more likely to enjoy yourself.

Sometimes it's hard to switch off and become sexual. During a sexual encounter anything and everything can get in the way, and women are more likely to be distracted by stray thoughts. To avoid this, practice relaxation and focus exercises. For example, jump into a cold

If you feel intimidated by the media portrayal of "sex kittens" turn to IDEA 47, *Hedonism*, to discover the real sex secrets of the Hollywood goddesses.

Try another idea...

swimming pool and relish the shock you feel in the first few seconds. Later think back to how your body felt and imagine giving over to just this sensation. Take this technique with you to the bedroom and concentrate on good physical sensations. Forget about the holy grail of orgasm. Think of it as a bonus, but that the scenic route, long and meandering, has its plus points, too.

Depression is linked to low libido, so downplay psychological issues that get in the way. Accept that sex is also a form of nonverbal communication and sometimes we use it to express other things, like saying "I'm sorry" or to express anger and frustration as well as tenderness. Don't fuss overly about how you look. Although the advertising industry wants you to believe that young and beautiful equals sexy, all the research indicates that the best sex is enjoyed by women over thirty. During World War I, the women who gave birth to the greatest number of illegitimate babies were in the thirty to thirty-five age group. Don't put too much emphasis on physical techniques until you've done the most important thing— adjusted your mind.

"Our sexuality doesn't make us who we are, but who we are affects the way our sexuality is understood by ourselves and others."
KATH ALBURY, author

Defining idea...

3

How did it go?

Q   Are some people naturally "better" at sex than others?

A   *It seems so. In 2005 geneticist Dr. Khytam Dawood published a study in
Twin Research that suggested a woman's ability to climax was partly due to
her genes. His team looked at more than 3,000 identical and nonidentical
twins and found that for 51 percent being able to successfully climax
through masturbation was due to genetic factors. However, their genes had
less of a role to play during sexual intercourse (31 percent) and other
methods (37 percent). As so little is known about how sexual arousal is
generated in the first place, we can only guess that being able to orgasm is
a combination of mental and physical factors. Dr. Marty Klein on libida.com
writes: "Desire = biology + psychology + relationship + culture + situation."*

**Q   I'm actually looking for practical tips to improve my sex life. Can
you help?**

A   *You'll find plenty of ideas for physical techniques and tricks, but don't
forget many women need to have some level of psychological arousal
before these can work. There are no universal, one-size-fits-all techniques
to rev up your sex life. Some people love G-spot–enhanced sex, others can't
feel it. Don't forget that every sex survey has some level of bias; often the
publicly funded ones are concerned with risk (teenage pregnancy,
transmission of STDs, and threats to marriage). Sex therapy tends to
emphasize performance over feelings, so concentrating on how you feel and
making a conscious effort to be more positive is the best start you can
make.*

2

Solo player

Being able to "get off" alone means more intense orgasms with someone else. One of the best ways to maintain your sex drive is to set regular pleasure sessions—with yourself.

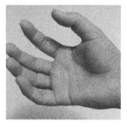

Having better orgasms means being able to put your finger on the right spot. If you know how to turn yourself on, you can point somebody else in the right direction.

Some feel a little dirty when they indulge, others finger themselves frantically in front of their partners, but sex researchers estimate that around 80 percent of women of all ages masturbate, and that means most of us are doing it.

Often in a stable relationship the frequency of masturbation sessions drops off. This is all well and good, but you can get into bad habits in bed and associate any negativity or frustration with the sex act itself. That's why it's crucial to be able to make yourself come satisfactorily—you can separate desire from the whole range of complex feelings you may have about your partner.

Here's an idea for you...

Before masturbating, try pressing your knees together and clenching your butt upward in rocking movements. This helps to stimulate the flow of blood to the general area—after a few minutes you should notice a difference in your vaginal sensations.

Self-pleasure is often rushed or abrupt. This may be a legacy of sneaky sessions under bedcovers from the time when you lived with your parents. In *The Illustrated Guide to Extended Massive Orgasm,* Steve and Vera Bodansky say that most people fail to take the best possible pleasure from masturbation because they "do it to relieve themselves" rather than for pleasure. I suggest practicing alone first so that you can experiment and work without expectations. Of course, you can add this to your lovemaking routine later.

How you prepare to masturbate is important. Some prefer to take advantage of the heat of the moment, or you might want to take a bath first, or perhaps dip into an erotic novel to get some saucy ideas. Don't dive straight in. By the time you undress you should feel pleasantly warm and stimulated. Experiment with what feels good, tease your nipples, run your hands over the whole pubic region.

Open your legs wide; the sensation of air should feel pleasant. It's best to wriggle your hips now and wait until your labia lips are swollen: this way they will swell, increasing sensitivity and moisture. Dip an exploratory finger just inside your vaginal lips; if you are wet, now is a good time to find out what turns you on. (If you are dry, then use a little lubricant like KY Jelly to get things running smoothly.) Use the dribble of moisture on your finger and run your finger around your vaginal lips. Feel for the outline of the labia majora (outer lips) and contrast this with your inner vagina (labia minora). You might want to experiment with the perineum—the skin between the vagina and the anus. Try circles, figure eights, and even tapping motions with your hand. What feels good? You should be nice and moist. Perhaps your clitoris is already retracting from its little hood of skin.

The most erotic part of your body is your mind. Perhaps you need to work on your fantasy life first; check out IDEA 20, *Mind games*.

Try another idea...

Now is a good time to explore your clitoris. Some women prefer to have one finger in the vagina while the other searches for the right spot. Feel for the clitoris and see which way and what type of strokes feel good. The clitoris is bigger than previously thought and has "arms" that are buried underneath the skin—experiment with the whole area to find your soft spot.

If it doesn't feel sensitive, try using your other hand to pull your skin away from the clitoris. At the same time, look for a second erogenous zone to maximize your pleasure. This could be a finger or two in the vagina, massaging your outer lips, or some form of anal stimulation. You might want to use a vibrator, anal butt plug, or some other toy to help you along.

Continue experimenting until you feel a peak, a point where it no longer feels intense. Rest and repeat.

Don't worry if you feel that the earth hasn't moved—we still haven't worked out how to describe the female orgasm. The urologist J. G. Bohlen found there was little difference between the perception of orgasm by women and physiological signs of it as measured in the laboratory.

"Masturbation: the primary sexual activity of mankind. In the nineteenth century it was a disease; in the twentieth, it's a cure."
THOMAS SZASZ, psychiatric specialist

Defining idea...

7

How did
it go?

Q   Whatever I do, I can't seem to find anything pleasurable about touching my clitoris. Is there something wrong with me?

A   *The short answer is no. A 1994 survey by the University of Chicago's National Opinion Research Center found that 10 percent of women don't experience orgasm at all, although once a woman learns how to do it she rarely loses the ability. For about one in ten women the vaginal lips have even more nerve endings than the clitoris. Other women have alternative hot spots, so don't worry if this isn't a crucial spot for you. Before trying again, try to stimulate yourself mentally first and touch your clitoris only when you are already in a state of arousal—you should feel wet and sticky. The clitoris is like a small bud, covered by a "hood" of loose skin, so take care to pull away its protective cover. Most women prefer the "ten to two" position, but you can try strokes, circles, or tapping to get the desired effect.*

Q   I've gone without sex so long the last thing I want to do is masturbate. Why should I try?

A   *You don't have to masturbate, it's up to you. Researchers have found that women who can successfully masturbate by themselves are much more likely to have more and better orgasms with someone else. You could go for a different sensation by putting an ice cube or the skin of a freshly peeled banana over the area to experience the feeling of sensory input. Experiment: find what feels good.*

3

Sticky fingers

What's what down there? Feel for the signs of your fertility; it might mean there are times when you feel extra sexy and days when it's just not happening.

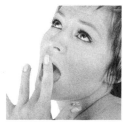

Understanding your body tunes you in to your natural cycle, tells you when you are most likely to get pregnant (or not), and can identify health problems. Over to you...

We're not talking about the rhythm method here—the problem with stuff like standard manuals and pregnancy wheels is that they cling to the myth of the twenty-eight day cycle with ovulation at day fourteen. In real life, women can ovulate from day eight to very late; less than 15 percent of cycles are twenty-eight days—a certain Dr. Rudi Vollman demonstrated the mean average cycle to be, in fact, twenty-nine and a half days—bad news if you're using the calendar method of contraception!

Be a step ahead and chart your fertility signs: vaginal mucus, waking temperature, and the position of the cervix. The primary sign (the easiest one to spot) is vaginal mucus, which changes as you progress through your cycle. After your period, mucus is dry or nonexistent. In the second week, as ovulation approaches, it becomes

Here's an idea for you...

Keep an "arousal" diary. Once a day, insert a finger into your vagina and check the moisture levels. Are you dry, wet, creamy, or slippery? Now compare your sexual activities. Did the changes in your vaginal environment affect your sexual enjoyment? If you can find a link, you'll be jumping over yourself to schedule sexual activity when you are most receptive.

wetter, and as ovulation nears, you release a slippery secretion, similar to sperm. This is designed as a sort of swimmable transport to get sperm to the egg and its role is crucial. One of the reasons why older women are less fertile is simply because they have fewer "egg white" days.

Many women feel sexier around the time they ovulate, thanks to the effects of estrogen which means, in Greek, "to make mad with desire." The wet sensation of the cervical fluid feels similar to the excited feeling of being "wet" although it's not the same as vaginal arousal. Cervical fluid comes from deep in the cervix, while arousal lubricant is a kind of sweat produced from the vaginal walls. For many women the second week of the month is the most interesting sexually for them and produces red-hot orgasms. On the downside, if you have sex during ovulation it's possible for your partner's penis to hit the follicle that is about to burst and release the egg—this can be eye-wateringly painful. You can also get mood swings and cramps, so pay attention to your calendar to find out if this is a hot time for you. If it is, time your encounters around the moments when you're likely to be more sensitive and have more satisfying orgasms.

Defining idea...

"Vagina is a totally ridiculous, unsexy word. It sounds like an infection at best, maybe a medical instrument: 'Hurry, Nurse, bring me the vagina.'"
EVE ENSLER

After ovulation, next comes the influence of progesterone, which turns your mucus sticky and creamy, literally plugging the cervix so any implantation can happen in peace. As you approach your period, the vagina becomes more acidic and itchy and more prone to infections (especially yeast), so this is the time where you might enjoy sex the least.

OK, you've been charting diligently, but something doesn't feel right. For the low-down on sensitive issues, head over to IDEA 29, _Ouch!_

Try another idea...

Some people simply make a note of their mucus changes (Billing's method). You can also take your waking temperature every day—it should rise _after_ you've ovulated because progesterone is a heat-inducing hormone. An optional added measure is to feel the shape of the cervix, which is softer and lower near ovulation. These methods are free, simple, and you can use these signs to plan better sex. If you know your vagina is more irritable just before your period, then this is when you do something other than have penetrative sex! It's also easier for you to detect real vaginal infections when they occur if you're charting, and erratic basal body temperatures can show thyroid or hormonal problems at an early stage. OK, you don't have to go the whole hog and don a white coat to perform this stuff, just think of it as an optional sextra that also helps you feel more comfortable with getting yourself off!

"It is amazing how few women really know what their external anatomy looks like. Sadly, most girls are led to believe that they are 'dirty down there,' and are therefore reluctant to examine themselves. Boys, however, are usually socialized to believe they possess a treasure in which to take pride."
TONI WESCHLER, fertility educator

Defining idea...

How did it go?

Q   I don't want to get pregnant—why should I worry about my cycle?

A   *Any long-term irregularities in your cycle ultimately lead to endometrial disease (cancer), and, unfortunately, something like ovarian cancer has a fatality rate of 80 percent within two years of diagnosis. Here's what Katie Singer, author of* A Guide to Charting Your Fertility Signals, *says about the general benefits of charting: "I began noticing that about 25 percent of the women who take my workshops are not ovulating. Or, their charts indicate that they may have hypothyroidism or progesterone deficiency. Often, more than one of these conditions shows up in the charts. Until they begin observing their fertility signals, most of these women consider themselves to be in good health. However, a woman who ovulates infrequently or not at all, for example, is at increased risk of uterine cancer, diabetes, polycystic ovarian syndrome, infertility, and other health problems." That seems like a lot of fringe benefits to get from a sticky finger!*

Q   I have a problem now that my boyfriend's moved away. We get together every couple of weeks and I'm a bit sore afterward. Any ideas?

A   *This is not really related to your cycle, although you may notice it worsens just before your period. Try to avoid "binge" sex, although it's pretty difficult in your case. Gynecologist Dr. Carol Livoti says in* Vaginas, An Owner's Manual: *"That's really not what the vagina is designed for. Inside, it's all thin mucous membranes, which are very delicate." Try to have sex more evenly rather than five times in one night; there are plenty of alternatives to rock your boat.*

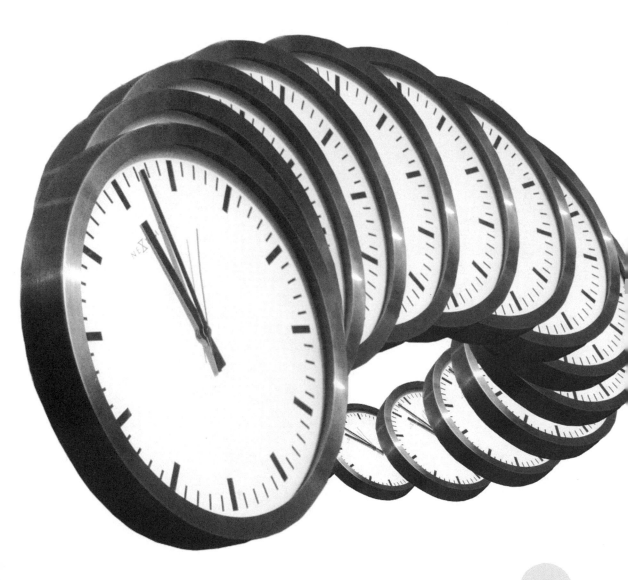

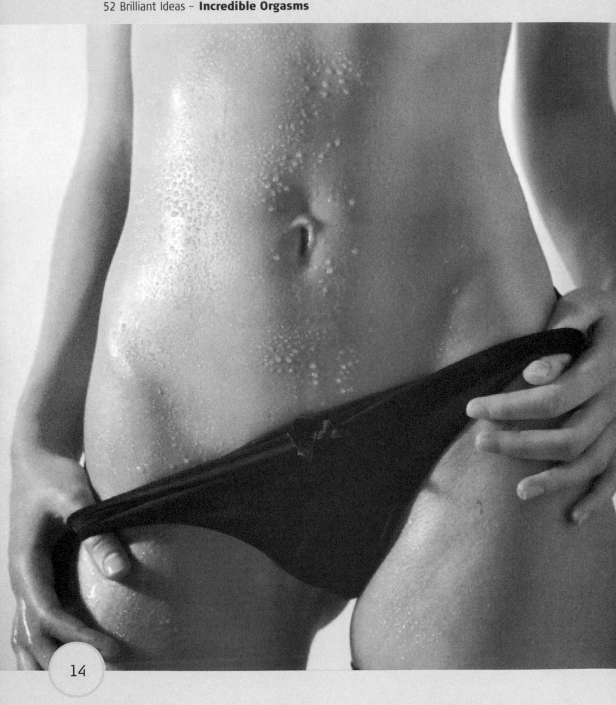

4

The beautiful and the bad

Seems as if only models and rock stars get good sex? Insecurity eats away at desire and anyone can have a hang-up.

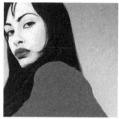

Don't let pictures of the beautiful and famous make you feel inadequate. Actually, the top performers, models, and stars probably feel more insecure than you do.

Beautiful women are held up as an ideal and yet top models, stars, and performers suffer more than you think. They seem to have it all—looks, public adoration, money—but the cult of celebrity often makes people more insecure. Success is fleeting and many stars are anxious about losing their status or plagued with self-doubt and addictions. Jib Fowles did a study in *Starstruck: Celebrity Performers and the American Public* that showed that celebrities are four times more likely to kill themselves than the average person.

And it's not just the pressures of fame. Even the most beautiful women can have problems feeling confident. Halle Berry is a former Miss Teen All America, was the runner-up to Miss USA, and has been voted into *People* magazine's Most Beautiful

Here's an idea for you...

Get some glamorous photographs taken of you (if necessary by a professional) and keep a few of them, framed, in your bedroom. This is to remind you that you are sexy, and the better the photo the more confidence you'll feel. After all, glam shots in magazines are hardly simple snapshots!

People list nine times: oh, and she's also an Oscar winner. Despite all this, she recently announced that she is very insecure about both her physical appearance and her acting. On Femalefirst.com she said, about those who pay her compliments: "If they really knew me, they'd realize I'm far from secure about my looks." Knowing that such a successful, talented, good-looking woman is plagued by self-doubts should convince you that beauty is skin deep. There's no point in thinking that you would feel/be sexier if you looked differently; confidence comes from within.

Similarly, Madonna, who is perhaps the most media-savvy female performer ever, has admitted, "I think my biggest flaw is my insecurity . . . I'm plagued with insecurities 24/7." In *Madonna: An Intimate Biography*, J. Randy Taraborrelli quotes dancer Sallim Gauwloos, who appeared in the movie *In Bed with Madonna*: "But she was very, very insecure, especially with other women. We would have parties, and there would never be beautiful women invited. Only guys. She would freak out if there was someone in the room more beautiful than her." Clearly, public persona and how stars really feel are two different things. Lesson learned—the grass is not greener on the other side.

One of the first supermodels of the late '70s, Gia Carangi, became a *Vogue* cover girl at eighteen and partied at New York's legendary Studio 54 with rock stars and royalty, but her spiraling fame left her unable to live up to her public image. By twenty-six she became one of the first American women to die of AIDS: her life story, *Thing of Beauty*, is not a pretty story.

You know you want to, so be adventurous and turn to IDEA 33, Let yourself go.

Try another idea...

Many regular women feel intimidated when they see airbrushed, perfect images of women in the media. Only 20 percent of American women are happy with their size; 50 percent of all women in the US are on a diet at any one time, although most of them are not even clinically overweight. In *The Body Project: An Intimate History of American Girls*, Joan Jacobs Brumberg says that girls' identities these days "revolve around the body rather than the mind, heart, or soul." We are just obsessed with how we look and having all this angst is a terrible burden on our sex lives.

In *Hot Monogamy*, Dr. Patricia Love uses research that shows women who have a negative body image are "less interested in making love . . . more restricted in their range of sexual activities, and have more difficulty becoming aroused and reaching orgasm." You have to feel sexy to have a better love life, rather than focusing on how you look. If you like, you can continue to feel down on yourself but it's better not to waste all that energy: concentrate instead on getting that orgasm high.

"A sex symbol becomes a thing. I hate being a thing."
MARILYN MONROE

Defining idea...

How did it go?

Q There have always been beautiful women on TV. Why all this focus on pretty women in the media?

A   *True, but today weight loss is a $50 billion per year industry in the US and the ideal of what we should look like is getting positively gaunt. As journalist Hazel Croft says: "In the 1950s models weighed 8 percent less than the average woman. In the 1990s models weighed 23 percent less. That makes models thinner than some 95 percent of the population." The difference between the ideal and the reality has never been further apart. Today there's so much more focus on how we look, people pierce their bodies, sculpt them with exercise, and are increasingly turning to cosmetic surgery. But what do they actually achieve by doing all this?*

Q Even knowing the insecurities of people like Halle Berry doesn't stop me from feeling jealous. Am I alone?

A   *No . . . there's a lot of it around. In a Nerve.com essay Lisa Gabriele is somewhat envious of Paris Hilton: "She's so thin and pliable, she should register her body as a font." If the overwhelming majority of us feel our bodies leave a lot to be desired, we're being our own worst enemies. Through sex we can learn to feel good about ourselves. Try masturbating more often and spending time naked; you need to get comfortable in your own skin.*

5

Slippery when wet

Different ways to get both your genitals glowing. Don't think prelude to penetration, savor it as the main event. Go on, take a chance!

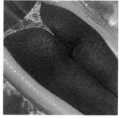

Play, touch, and intimacy are just as vital to foreplay as mastery of the basic sexual techniques. Tease each other and don't worry about going all the way.

There's no right way to do foreplay because everyone has a different sexual "script" of what turns them on, and what we feel like on Monday might not be the same thing we're in the mood for on Tuesday. The only way to indicate your preferences is to communicate, using your voice and body language—or even flaunting an established signal, such as wearing a particular dress or shade of lipstick that has become codified to indicate something naughty.

Ideally, touching and intimacy should be part of your relationship and not just restricted to the bedroom. Couples who are touchy-feely massage and cuddle each other while doing other things like watching TV and chatting to friends, and if you relish the touch of your lover at any time you're likely to move more quickly on to sexual play. Get your partner to be considerate of you in little things like tidying up

Hang a sheet up in the middle of a room (or from a coat hanger on your wardrobe door) and stand on either side of it so that you can't see each other. Naked, feel for each other through the sheet and rub lightly up against each other. What you think about during this, I'll leave to you. The novelty of the experience should make you feel aroused more quickly.

after himself; some psychologists think foreplay is the combined effect of your partner's behavior long before any sex takes place. Aline P. Zoldbrod says in *Sex Talk:* "... There is something crucial before physical foreplay. It is all of the talking and actions that have happened during the last twelve hours or so of togetherness."

The secret to good foreplay is to stop seeing it as a prelude to intercourse. When we start a new relationship we spend a lot more time kissing, hugging, and touching, and we should be able to indulge in this at any time without needing to go all the way. Play around a little and find out what gets each other off. Get your partner to talk dirty to you, moan more, or indicate with his hands which spots feel good and, likewise, point him in the right direction. It could be that you just love having your toes sucked, your neck bitten, or your bottom spanked, but the only way to find out is to have lots of practice. It's actually more exciting if you get into the habit of playing around, with no pressure to reach orgasm or move on to penetrative sex; that way, each occasion keeps you both guessing. A lot of couples get into a kind of linear foreplay—first he feels your breasts, kisses you, and then moves down south, and after approximately five minutes you assume the missionary position. Sex doesn't

"Too much of a good thing is wonderful."
MAE WEST

have to be routine. Feel free to change the order in which you do things and to move from penetration to oral sex. Don't be afraid to lend a hand and play with yourself in front of him, too.

On average, we devote around twenty minutes to foreplay, according to the Durex 2004 Global Sex Survey. If your partner rushes things, play around while you are still fully clothed. Rubbing yourself against his hard crotch through your jeans can feel magnificent, and when he touches you it'll feel better if you're already hot. Before you get to naked genital contact, try kissing, light touches (with fingertips or feathers), and breast and neck play. He could try cupping your genitals with one hand while the other presses on your pubic bone. If you like oral sex, try it in different positions; for instance, receiving it while in the doggy position feels completely different than lying on your back. If your partner is licking/kissing you, he can also try varying from hot/cold temperatures or sucking a mint or cough lozenge, all of which will change how his tongue feels.

Play around a little and don't be afraid to introduce sex toys. Whatever you do, keep it fun and sexy. You know what they say, sometimes it's more fun to travel than to arrive!

Many women find it easier to get aroused by oral sex: see IDEA 7, *Get him to use his mouth.*

Try another idea...

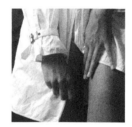

"The sexual embrace can only be compared with music and with prayer."
HAVELOCK ELLIS, author and researcher

Defining idea...

How did it go?

Q   How long should it take for me to get aroused during foreplay?

A   There is no set time, although Dr. Ian Kerner says in his book She Comes First *that if their partner spends at least twenty-one minutes on foreplay, 92.3 percent of women are guaranteed an orgasm. His results, though, are based on a small sample. Other women need much more or less than this. Women over thirty-five tend to prefer less foreplay, whereas men of the same age are likely to want more (men need more stimulation as they get older to maintain an erection). Many women complain they don't get enough foreplay, but it could be that their partners are doing what they think turns them on and not what actually does. Tell him what you want. To slow him down, find nongenital ways of stimulating him, such as rubbing his perineum or massaging his stomach.*

Q   Why do men get aroused so much more quickly than women?

A   Perhaps because a penis is so much more of a hands-on piece of anatomy. A man knows he's aroused when his penis is hard, but often women have no physical clue. Being wet doesn't mean you're aroused, as vaginal lubrication depends on where you are in your cycle and what medications you're taking. Researchers have also found that a lot of foreplay is led by the male partners, so use a bit of girl power!

6

Shivering with anticipation

Just the thought of your new lover or favorite fantasy can make you wet. Charge yourself up into an erotic good mood.

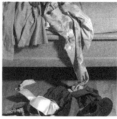

Thinking dirty thoughts might seem like the easiest thing in the world, but a lot of us have problems getting there, so you need to examine the most intimate connections of your mind.

How you get emotionally psyched up into feeling sexy is a very personal thing; in fact scientists know very little about the relationship between arousal and erotic connection. Some experiments have been carried out, mostly with male animals like rats and quail. Like Pavlov's dogs, certain responses can be conditioned, but females (whether animals or human) respond less to external stimuli. The main problem Hoffmann, Janssen, and Turner found in a 2004 study on classic conditioning and sexual arousal was that the conditioning could occur on a subliminal basis, with the participants unable to recall the picture their bodies had responded to. This means that we may be unaware of the very erotic connection

Get into the habit of writing down your dreams. When you go to sleep, think erotic thoughts and hopefully you'll have raunchy dreams all night—which will mean you'll wake up feeling wet and ready for a bit of love. The more you can train yourself to think sexy at odd times, like when you're waiting in a supermarket line, the faster you'll be able to perform when it really counts.

that arouses us, making it extra difficult for us to use conscious visualization techniques to get in the mood.

The simple solution is that we have to try harder. If you're having problems getting going, think back and remember a time when you had great sex and try to get into that mindset. For me, the sight of a ripe, golden cornfield is always sensuous; it takes me back to the heady days of being twelve, under the thrall of my first crush. Try to put yourself on the couch and think about what situations are erotic for you. Or create new scenarios where you imagine yourself getting turned on. Most erotic images are narcissistic and show poses with models whose bodies effectively say "Look at me." It's rare to actually see someone captured in the throes of orgasm, carried away by their passions. Don't think about how you look, concentrate on how it feels. Use the same covert rehearsal techniques that athletes use to psych themselves up for competitions. If you visualize yourself having a wonderful sexual experience, right down to the expression on your face and the perspiration dripping as you climax, it's much more likely to happen. Positive thinking and sexual self-confidence are the most useful tools we can arm ourselves with.

Another trick is to devote a little time to just thinking about sexy thoughts: for instance, giving yourself a chance to daydream, to browse erotica, and the freedom to respond to sexual imagery. In a Xandria.com article, Betty Dodson suggests we tap into our aural pleasure because we've been conditioned to climax and have sex silently. She recommends recording an orgasm with a tape recorder/dictaphone and playing it back; you'll probably find it's more subdued than you realize. Just practicing coming in a louder, sexier way can help to free your inhibitions.

To examine yourself more closely, turn to IDEA 1, *What sexual thoughts are you made of?*

Try another idea...

Many couples try to pep up a flagging sex life with more foreplay. However, there is something crucial that needs to occur before manual attempts at stimulation: we need to open our minds and psych ourselves up to eagerly anticipate sexual adventures. Clinical psychologist Peggy J. Kleinplatz, in a Womanspirit.net article, cites a case where the female patient finds arousal easy when she masturbates, but experiences difficulty with her partner: "She says that the problem is that he touches her genitals in order to arouse her, prior to intercourse, but that there is no use in touching her genitals until she is sexually aroused. How does she become aroused? She becomes aroused in response to either non-genital touch or to the sense of erotic connection." It's this mental spark that we need to cultivate, the elusive je ne sais quoi that captivates our erotic imagination.

Lovers should spend time talking, thinking, imagining, and reveling in each other's possibilities before moving on to manual techniques. It really is a question of mind over matter!

"Eroticism can override an awful lot of lousy technique. In fact, erotic connection can generate sexual excitement in the absence of any physical contact at all."
PEGGY J. KLEINPLATZ, psychologist

Defining idea...

25

How did
it go?

Q   So are you saying that women need longer to get turned on than men?

A   *Not always. Women tend to be faster at getting there through masturbation.* Jonathan Margolis notes in O: The Intimate History of the Orgasm, *"Women can normally masturbate from stone cold to orgasm in about four minutes. Men, however, as women do in 'real' sex, often need to get into the mood either by careful mental scene setting, or the visual stimulus of pornography . . ."* Despite this, most women prefer sex with someone else to autoeroticism. Our strength is that we are more "erotically plastic," but this makes it harder to condition ourselves to new sexual behavior like, for instance, the particular lovemaking style of a new partner.

Q   Is there something wrong with me if I'm slow to get mentally turned on?

A   *No.* Therapist Peggy J. Kleinplatz thinks that we focus too much on the mechanics of getting an erect penis and lubricated vagina. She thinks sex therapy concentrates on the mechanics of desire rather than the cognitive erotic connections that generate it in the first place. She also points out that the "norm" sex therapists work toward "involves two, able-bodied heterosexuals in a monogamous relationship." Don't worry about being different. Kleinplatz says, "We may have a great deal to learn from/about the farther reaches of human sexuality if we quit pathologizing what seems alien and embrace it instead."

7

Get him to use his mouth

Think original sin, Eve, and that symbolic snake.
Astounding and wonderful things to have done to you . . .

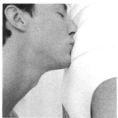

Being able to enjoy oral sex, as a starter or an act in itself, is a good way to ensure you have satisfying orgasms. Many women find it easier to come this way than during penetrative sex.

First, you can't get the full benefits if you're worried about how you will look and taste when he gets up close and personal. A healthy vagina is actually cleaner than the mouth and has the same odor and taste as natural yogurt. Even if it's been hours since your last shower, it'll still taste OK after a few licks. We probably obsess too much about personal hygiene; by all means take a relaxing bath or shower beforehand, but remember that recently applied soap may taste just as odd. A quick rinse with water is a great freshener.

And don't worry about how your vagina looks—your partner does not have eyes in his tongue! Models in porn get a lot of work done down there, including plastic surgery and liposuction as well as makeup, so become comfortable with yourself in front of a mirror before you get into scenes with a partner.

Treat yourself to a pair of real silk undies and get your partner to spend as long as possible licking you through the material before he gets to your clit. When you've been teased and tingled for a while you'll be screaming for more.

Feeling relaxed is the best state to be in when he goes down on you. A good trick is to start with all-over kissing. You can also check for beard stubble; is it too rough on your flesh? Now is a good time to sort out hand signals so you can maneuver him properly on your pleasure center. You want the full works, don't you? That's right, don't lie there passively. Ask him to tease you around the inner thighs and to kiss your legs and belly. If someone dives straight in, use your hands to push him gently away. Give him a hand by opening your vaginal lips with your hands. Feel free to warm up by playing with your clitoris. The more aroused you are before the tongue gets there, the hotter it will feel!

If you already know what tongue techniques you like best, indicate this to your partner by licking his hand in the same motion. Lie down on your back, preferably at the end of a sofa or on a bed with a pillow under your butt. Use your hands to guide your partner's head. Many women like to be subjected to teasing of the outer vulva and inner thighs first. Your partner should be able to see signs of you becoming aroused—such as a reddening and swelling of the inner lips as well as an increase in vaginal lubrication. You may like sucking, licking, or

Defining idea...

"If he is queasy about oral sex, then you definitely need to know, because . . . it's a very important part of you—a part of you that needs satisfaction as much as your partner's penis does."
VIOLET BLUE, sex educator

mild biting on specific areas, but don't let your partner blow into the vagina as this can create air embolism (it can be fatal—not good).

When you are fully stimulated, you may be ready for direct action on the clitoris. It has an astonishing 8,000 nerve endings despite having no real job or function, so it can be a bit intense. Nifty tongue circles around it work well, so get your partner to try figure eights and playful flicks in an up and down or left to right movement. Some women like the tongue to dart in and out of the vagina, others like a finger in the vagina or anus while the clitoris is being attended to. This heightens the sexual feeling because the pleasure areas overlap. Some clitorises are more sensitive on one side; use your mouth to scream where. It should feel amazing by now!

When it does feel good, give yourself time for the pleasure to build. Some lie still, others grind their hips in motion. Do whatever works for you. Some people like to straddle the face of the person licking them so they have complete control. Surrender yourself freely to the experience and give your partner the thrill of feeling that gush of final wetness as you come.

If you're concerned about the size or appearance of your vagina, check out IDEA 11, *The long and short of it*, for reassurance.

Try another idea…

"Make sure you kiss someone before you go to bed with him. Pay careful attention. Does he thrust his tongue down your throat as if he's searching for the Holy Grail? Does he mash his teeth against your lips? If so, drop him flat."
CYNTHIA HEIMEL, author

Defining idea…

How did it go?

Q   **Although many of my friends have oral sex, it's something my mother won't even mention. Why the sudden interest in this activity?**

A   *They say there's nothing new under the sun. There's oral sex on pottery from 300 BC and lots of it going on in the* Kama Sutra, *written in AD 400. Animals routinely sniff and taste each other's bits so we can guess that humans have always been doing the same. In* Sperm Wars: The Science of Sex *biologist Robin Baker suggests that oral sex is an opportunity to gather information about a partner's reproductive health and check for signs of any recent infidelity! The odd thing is that Eastern countries that were previously liberal have adopted the Western, post-Victorian aversion to sex. Jonathan Margolis, in* O: The Intimate History of the Orgasm, *says, "Some of the world's most abbreviated foreplay occurs in rural China, where 34 percent of couples are now said to spend less than a minute on sexual preamble and oral sex is almost unknown, the modern Chinese, even in sophisticated cities, regarding it as 'too dirty.'" Sexual attitudes are like fashion, they go in and out!*

Q   **How can I have safer oral sex?**

A   *If you are not "fluid bonded" you can use gloves (for fingers) and dental dams—small squares of latex that are quite thick. Worst-case scenario: cut up a condom or use plastic wrap.*

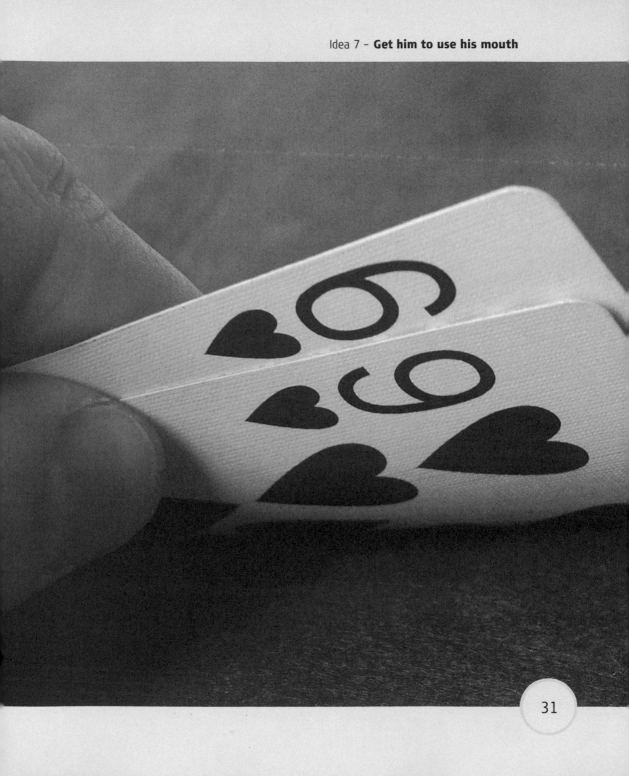

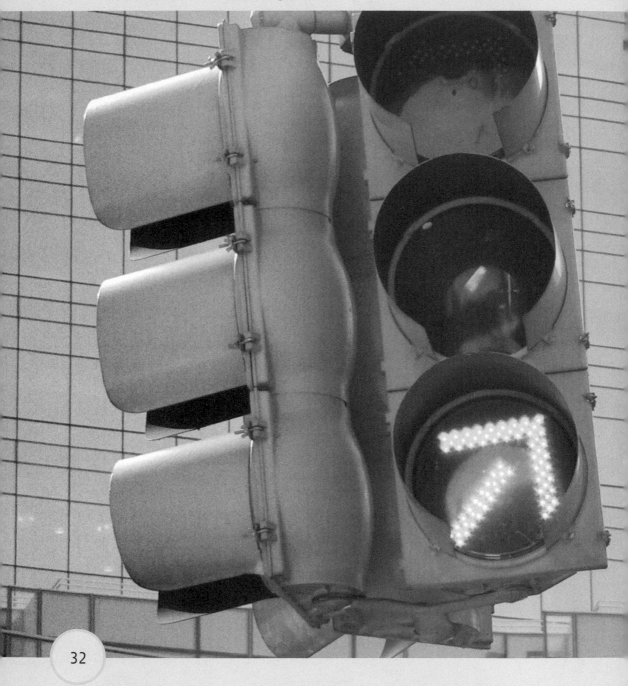

8

Starter's orders

Men and women can get equally aroused, just not at the same time. It's a bitch, but you've got to get the timing right.

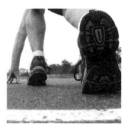

Ways to slow down the pace and get your partner to be more touchy-feely...

The Kinsey studies on sexuality in 1939 and 1950 revealed basic sex behavior differences that remain unchanged despite drastic changes in our lifestyles. Contemporary researchers were surprised to find that although women have more sexual partners, masturbate more, and have more oral sex, they are still more likely than men to have gaps in their sexual activity, experience arousal difficulties, and prefer sex in a committed relationship. When women decide to be excited, they can get aroused as easily as men but their desire is generated differently. In *What Women Want—What Men Want*, John Marshall Townsend says, "But the cues for her arousal are initially internal: she must put herself in the mood, or allow herself to be put in the mood."

Being able to get in the mood for sex is crucial, so tell your partner the things that help you get to that special place. Men and women are simply different sexually: men are more likely to respond to visual stimuli, but women prefer touching and

Here's an idea for you...

Ask your partner to give you some time alone to get in the mood, anything from ten to thirty minutes, but don't agree on what time he should come in and disturb you. Start to masturbate; the fact that you don't know when to expect him will add to your tension. Let him catch you playing with yourself, and when he sees what you're up to you should be already nicely aroused.

behavior that suggests an emotional investment. Men often dive right in to genital play because that's what they prefer, but if you're into some romantic kissing first, followed by breast fondling, then simply keep kissing him until he gets the message and slow foreplay down to a tempo that you're comfortable with.

If you're already naked and he's too eager, try one of the tips from the *Kama Sutra*—the Biting of a Boar. He sits on his haunches and you sit between his knees with your back to him. He can kiss or lightly bite (or breathe on) your back, shoulders, and neck. Another move is the Kiss that Awakens, when you lie down on your stomach and pretend to be prettily asleep while he kisses your neck, ears, back, cheeks, and lips in order to awaken you.

Defining idea...

"Writing is like making love. Don't worry about the orgasm, just concentrate on the process."
ISABEL ALLENDE

If he's too eager, avoid genital contact because this will make him want to climax even more urgently. Instead, massage his perineum or buttocks or another area of his body. Once a man is fully aroused he can reach the point of "ejaculatory inevitability" when it becomes imperative for him to come—quickly. To stave this off, you could start emotional foreplay earlier (before his mind has even started thinking about sex). Another tactic is to reward him for prolonging foreplay by performing a sexual treat that you know he enjoys. Another trick is to act like a dominatrix: some force their male clients to control their erections by making them wear a chastity belt, like the Stallion Guard, that inhibits erection. He'll probably find these methods of physical restraint alluring and it means you've got him under lock and key for as long as you like.

For tips on positions that help you to climax simultaneously, see IDEA 12, *Supersize it*.

Try another idea...

If he's prone to premature ejaculation or just too impatient, another approach is to get him to have a quick climax first so that he'll be able to focus on pleasing you. I once heard of a fetish club where each man received a blow job when he got through the door so he could properly enjoy the night's proceedings. If you don't feel like doing this, you can encourage him to masturbate, or do it for him using lots of lube. This will mechanically slow him down for his next orgasm because his seminal vesicle and prostate need time to create more seminal fluid.

If you reward each other with sexual treats you encourage positive reinforcement, and a study by Birnbaum, et al., in 2001 showed that consistent orgasms are associated with greater love for a partner and the feeling of being loved in return. Despite our preferences for a different tempo, we can still get it on.

"The power to charm the female has sometimes been more important than the power to conquer other males in battle."
CHARLES DARWIN

Defining idea...

How did
it go?

Q   **Is it natural to need so much foreplay?**

A   *Yes. Although some men have problems getting aroused, statistically men are quicker off the draw. Some ancient religions acknowledge this. In Ancient China followers of the Tao revelled in their partner's yin and a man was taught to feel his woman's nine erotic zones and five beautiful qualities. According to Geraldine Brooks in* Nine Parts of Desire, *Mohammed encouraged female sexuality: "When any one of you has sex with his wife, then he should not go to her like birds; instead you should be slow and delaying." In a 2004 study of 8,000 African-American women,* Ebony *magazine found that 56 percent of respondents said they'd like more foreplay and touching before and after intercourse.*

Q   **Isn't all this talk of men and women being different just cultural conditioning?**

A   *No. Researchers who looked at single, married, gay, lesbian, and heterosexual couples found the same basic patterns regardless of status or sexual orientation. In* O: The Intimate History of the Orgasm *Jonathan Margolis comments sardonically, "The genius of the genus is that the huge majority of us are not homosexual—that, for one reason or another, the complex attraction of otherness has always managed to outweigh the easy pleasures of sexual like-mindedness, and the furtherance of the species has thus been assured."*

9

Point of entry

Who wants to go first? The politics of penetration: Does your partner want to be the one and only dominator?

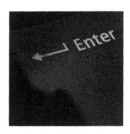

Daring ways to take the lead in seduction and play games of role-reversal for a bit of role bending!

Foreplay and sex are typically "led" by the man, especially penetration, which can leave women feeling like passive recipients. If women are slow to initiate sex, men have more anxiety because they have the pressure of sexually proving themselves and working out what women want. Simply by taking the lead in seduction, you can change the dynamics of your relationship.

Try focusing on him for a change and ask him to guide your hand in the right direction. Getting him to open up to what feels good is an excellent way to learn how to read each other's needs. See if he likes having his nipples played with and put an exploratory finger in his mouth to get him used to the feeling of being penetrated. This is all gentle stuff to get him used to the idea.

Take it in turns to take command of who does what in your lovemaking. When it's your turn, try something different and see if you can roll around from one position to the next. You can also choose a new position from fun websites like www.sexualpositionsfree.com— it uses only dolls in various poses, so you won't find it shocking.

Even if you elect for the missionary position, you can still become the active partner by initiating intercourse. Tell him when to insert his penis, or better still, make him go halfway and then withdraw, or wait. If you go for the more obvious woman on top position, move his body into the way you want it to show him you're in control.

An ingenious device to assist with positioning is getting a "love swing" fixed to the ceiling. This allows you to try a greater range of positions at angles that are just not possible lying on a bed. You can both sit on it, or one of you can lie spread-eagled, or hang tantalizingly over the edge. It also swings and bounces when you have sex and the movement intensifies the rhythm of your strokes. If you position your man on a love swing, you will increase his sense of helplessness.

This is an ideal place to do anal play on him. Try massaging the perineum first before tipping down to the anus. Trickle a bit of lube over it; you don't have to go any further yet, but let him get used to the feeling of being dominated. If he's interested, you could try gently inserting a finger or using an anal butt plug to keep him stimulated while you've got his whole body to play with. If he is responsive, then here's your chance to tease him with your own sex toy collection. Gently prod him with a

"Sex is an emotion in motion."
MAE WEST

38

dildo along his body (some men enjoy having it inserted in their mouth or anus) but first get him used to revering a phallic-shaped object in the way he likes you to worship his penis. This gives him a taste of how it feels when the roles are reversed. Don't forget that he might enjoy the buzz of a vibrator on his nipples and testicles, and he might even request that you put it in somewhere more intimate!

To go a step further, try using a strap-on harness. It's easier to get one fitted, so go to a good sex shop and ask for help. You can also buy a vibrating dildo that gives you sensations, too. Don't forget to warm him up with some light anal play first and to use lots of lube. Ask him to help you to penetrate by holding his anus more open. Take it slow and relish the feeling of being in control. Many men find it easier to identify with their partners after undergoing this experience. With practice you'll learn you can switch into a more dominant role whatever your position, which helps you to make the most of your sexual experiences.

For an alternative approach to sex, explore Eastern mysticism in IDEA 45, *Asian secrets*.

Try another idea...

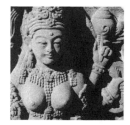

"Positioning is important. It says a lot about you—your political position, professional position, financial position, social position. But what about your sexual position?"
DR. SUSAN BLOCK, sex therapist

Defining idea...

How did
it go?

Q   I feel uncomfortable about taking the lead in bed. Is this usual?

A   *Many woman do, which is fine if you're having wonderful orgasms, but you could be missing out because you haven't had a chance to develop your sexual identity. In* Yes Means Yes, *Kath Albury says, "If women are raised to believe that sex is 'for men,' and this belief is confirmed by lackluster sexual experiences where her partner simply expects her to 'do her duty,' 'play along,' or 'prove she's not frigid,' then there's not much chance of her ever developing her own sexual desires." The trick is to start with slow steps; it's up to you how far you experiment.*

Q   Isn't all this male anal play a bit perverse?

A   *Many people, including heterosexual, gay, and lesbian couples, enjoy anal play. There's nothing "gay" about it; it doesn't indicate a preference for men, just enjoyment when stimulated anally. In a Queendom.com poll, men were asked if it turned them on to have their anal region stimulated and only a quarter answered no or not at all. The other three-quarters responded by choosing "enormously," "quite a bit," or "somewhat," so I guess that answers your question. The female respondents answered similarly, too. If you really want to get into the swing of it, invest in some toys and watch a girl-on-boy anal video like* Bend Over Boyfriend.

10

Classic positions

How do you do with those old favorites? You know—the ones you're sure even your mom knows.

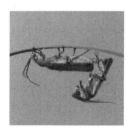

These classic sexual moves are here to stay, so make the most of them and modify them slightly for a little diversity...

Couples who experiment generally have a sexual repertoire that includes two or three basic positions, and these are likely to be the missionary, woman on top, and doggy style. It's often easier to begin sex play with missionary because with the woman prone on her back and the man's weight supported on his knees, it's an easier vantage point to actually insert the penis. If the man lies flat down on his partner, her pelvic movements are restricted, so he should rest more weight on his knees and lift his pelvis up so that she can rub her clitoris against his pelvic bone. For deeper penetration she can lift her legs up as far as possible, all the way to putting them over his shoulders. The higher you can get them back, the deeper the penetration.

For other variations, interlock your legs or twist them around his back to squeeze him tighter. An alternative is to close your legs to make the vaginal passage narrower. As with all sexual positions, it's not the posture but the way that you move to the strokes that creates the biggest difference in sensation. In *Satisfaction*

Here's an
idea for
you...
Get into the missionary position then try moving the position of your knees/legs. Can you bring them forward, lift them onto his legs? Changing your leverage makes all the difference. If he supports himself on his knees you can raise your lower body and, ironically, this position puts you in control.

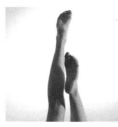

Kim Cattrall and Mark Levinson give advice about strokes: "A man tends to think in a linear way—that is, in and out. A woman tends to experience in a circular way—around and around. A penis going straight in and out of the vagina may lead to mutual satisfaction, but it tends to be much more effective when coupled with motions that reflect an arc or a circle." From this position, it's also easy to roll into sex sideways or (if you're adventurous) you can do a complete body roll so that you are upright in the next popular position, woman on top.

Both men and women generally find it easier to come when they're on top, and if you're pregnant or nervous about the depth of the penetration, being in control means that you take charge of the strokes. It's up to you whether to go for full penetration or just to play with the tip of the penis. For this reason it's a useful position for a woman who's never had sex before. You can lie down over your partner, balancing your weight forward onto your clitoris, and you're in an ideal position to use your knees to rock, thrust, or push your way to orgasm. You can also sit up (note that you get better penetration if you do this sitting on a chair with no arms so your legs can use the floor for leverage) and just choose to rock back and forth. A variation is to lean back more, still straddling his penis so your clitoris is exposed, making it easy for you to play with it and giving him a ringside seat. Another trick is for you to sit the other way, facing his feet reverse "cowgirl" style, which gives you a different feeling again and is ideal for men who worship an exposed derriere in action.

Doggy style or rear entry feels more animalistic. The emphasis is on penetration (it'll make his penis seem bigger) although he can use a deft hand to stimulate your clitoris and breasts at the same time. This one makes it easier for him to come, so often it's the explosive finale. You can either lie prone on your stomach or on all fours with the weight on your knees. His legs can be inside or outside yours; an alternative is to do it on your sides lying down.

Revisit these classic positions and put a little more *oomph* into them. It's easy and you won't need to look at a diagram while you're at it!

For better clitoral stimulation try the specially adapted positions in IDEA 12, Supersize it.

Try another idea...

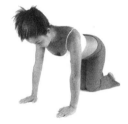

"Saying that missionary sex is your favorite is kind of like saying that you like bread a whole lot. Sure, everyone likes it, but it's not something you spent a great deal of time thinking about or that you need to form an opinion on."
REBECCA ARCHER, couples therapist

Defining idea...

How did it go?

Q   Is the missionary position really so popular?

A   Yes. Anthropologist Helen Fisher points out that the missionary position is, universally, the favored position in most cultures. There's a reason for that; although some see it as boring and old-fashioned, being able to do it is part of what makes us uniquely human—we've evolved with all our erogenous zones down our fronts to encourage us to adopt face-to-face sex. Doing it this way is friendly, allows sensuous full body contact, and gives us plenty of opportunity to gaze into each other's eyes. And we do it a lot, the author Ann Semans reckons: "Over 85 percent of married couples engage in the missionary position exclusively," so don't feel that you have to do an outlandish position to have great sex.

Q   I like the woman-on-top position, but I feel awkward initiating it. Any ideas?

A   You could try rolling onto your sides and having sex in this position for a while first before you roll over and get to be on top. Or you could sit on a table while your lover penetrates you standing up. Better still, sit your lover on a specially designed Hot Box from loving-angles.com and play with him a little bit first before jumping on top. This way you just sit on his lap rather than having to crawl over on a bed.

44

11

The long and short of it

**Just how important is size? Painful or not enough *oomph*?
Consider these variations for a better fit.**

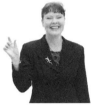

To some women penis size does matter; it can be too small or big. But other things also count: skin color, smell, and even the appearance of veins. In other words, it's not just about how long, how hard, and how thick.

Have you ever realized why showing an erect penis is taboo in most countries? Bernie Zilbergeld in *The New Male Sexuality* says it's because it's *men* who have penis envy. Men have few opportunities to compare themselves with regular erect penises (porn stars are almost always freakishly endowed), so a lot of them don't really know how they measure up. Poor things! That means it's usually girlfriends and wives who get to tell them how it really is.

Yep, this puts you in a position of power, but don't forget that having sex with someone once or even a couple of times doesn't make you an expert on how they are in bed. It takes a lot of practice to become tuned in to each other, which is why humans uniquely have around an eighteen-month "honeymoon" period when they

Here's an idea for you...

For a fuller feeling, try using an anal plug while having sex. This will help to shorten the vaginal opening because your perineum (the bit in the middle between your vagina and anus) is being pulled in two different directions. Kind of naughty but nice, it will also feel like you're having two men at once!

can't keep their hands off each other: about the time needed for prehistoric man to get a bun in the oven.

We're an average bunch, though. The Lifestyles Condom Penis Size survey measured 300 stiff penises and concluded (amazingly) that 82 percent of women were content with an average-sized penis of about 6 inches. Conveniently, it just so happens the average erect love stick is 5.9 inches and its girth 5 inches. Only 2 percent of women wanted an extra-large penis (over 10 inches, like you see in porn films) and only 9 percent wanted a bigger-than-average penis (7–8 inches). The "barrel" size of our vaginas also varies enormously and will change in size after giving birth, but it's only a mere 3–4 inches long, and the hidden G-spot is just 3 inches in. It just so happens that the vaginal entrance is more sensitive than the inner two-thirds: all good news for non-large men. However, during sex the inner two-thirds of the vagina expand and it lengthens/widens. Don't worry, as the vagina balloons the first part of it contracts and gives the friction there more frisson; non-mammoth penises have every chance to get the job done.

Defining idea...

Mae: "How tall are you?"
Man: "Six foot seven."
Mae: "Well, let's forget about the six foot and talk about the seven inches."
MAE WEST

Remember if you're a woman who's not had it in a while, you could be unusually excited and very wet, and end up with a lot of bumping and slipping. Solution—tissue off your excess juices. In some cultures a "dry" vagina is highly prized, and women use various potions and powders for an abrasive rub. However, most men will—and should—delight in a wet partner.

If you want more sensation, some positions are better suited for a smaller to average penis. The missionary position is improved with a pillow under the woman's bottom. Even better, if you can, bend your legs back and hook them around his neck. In *Supersex,* Tracey Cox says crossing your ankles in this position helps to tighten the vaginal canal. You'll also find that woman on top positions work well, especially if you sit on a chair so you have more leverage. Other favorites are doggy style (although some men report falling out); here, the best thing is for the man to use his hands to hold the woman's hips and control both thrusts. Others swear by the scissor position, lying with your heads in opposite directions, "scissoring" your legs with each other's (one of you has a leg underneath the other), and with you facing him in a sideways twist, holding hands.

Some men are too big for their partners. If this is the case it's better for you to be on top because you have more control or you can ask him to use only part of his penis to stimulate you until you feel ready for more. Use lots of lubricant to ease things along and most of all, whatever size you are, have fun!

The good news is that less well-endowed penises are easier to manipulate during oral sex, and are just perfect for anal sex: see IDEA 14, Alternative erogenous zones.

Try another idea...

"Every woman has a different comfort zone regarding penetration, and personal preferences range from a-pinky-at-most to king-sized-is-best."
CATHY WINKS, author

Defining idea...

How did
it go?

Q **After having my second child, my husband's penis feels like a
finger. What can we do to improve our sex life?**

A   *The short-term solution is to use some kind of sexual aid, while long term
you practice Kegel–pelvic floor–exercises to get back some of your muscle
tone. When he is inside you, can you insert a finger into your vagina? If so,
a good love aid is the penis girth extender, a set of pliant silicone inserts he
simply inserts along with his penis. You can also experiment with different
positions, and don't be afraid to use sex toys.*

Q **Although I'm happy with my partner, he's obsessed with the size
of his penis, which he thinks is too small. Do products like penis
pumps really work?**

A   *Men always want to have a bigger, thicker penis, but don't forget the
disadvantage of being well-endowed is that it's more difficult to get fully
hard (you need more blood in the area) and to stay that way. Penis pumps
can make a penis temporarily bigger because they suck more blood in, but
it doesn't last long and as sex therapist Dr. R. Williams says, "You run the
risk of getting lymph blisters on the glans of your penis from the
contraption you're putting over it." There's also the risk of burst capillaries
and temporary impotence, none of which sounds like a good Friday night.*

12

Supersize it

You know where it is and you want to feel it squirm. Some positions work extra hard to stimulate your clitoris. Try the CAT and the PUSSY and see if you meow.

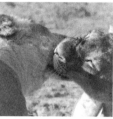

There's nothing acrobatic or difficult about the CAT and you could improve your chances of having an orgasm with it by up to 50 percent!

The best sex position for you is simply the one that feels best when you're doing it. Hopefully you've explored your own body and have gotten to know your top erogenous zones. Do you enjoy clitoral or G-spot stimulation? Some women feel more sensitive on their vaginal lips or perineum, or you may need a combination of different stimulations to get you off. You need to find the right position and angle, and work out what speed, pace, and rhythm works best, which are a lot of factors to get right in one try.

Many women need a lot of clitoral stimulation, but traditional sexual techniques often stimulate the vaginal area more, leaving some women extremely frustrated. To remedy this, the CAT (Coitally Adjusted Technique) was "invented" in the 1990s and it's specifically designed for extra clitoral stimulation. You start off in the basic missionary position, but your partner should rest his full weight on your chest and

Here's an idea for you...

Create your own new sex position. Experiment with postures and try moving your legs and pelvis differently for a better fit. The dominant person should try different ways of supporting their hands—higher, lower and prone on the body. Both of you have a chance at being on top and see whether you prefer to lean forward (for clitoral stimulation) or backward to nudge your G-spot.

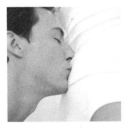

you should maneuver until you're lying with both pelvic bones touching. This way he's riding higher than normal (his forehead will be around six inches farther up the bed), most of his penis is out of your vagina, but the head of it is pressing alluringly against your clitoris. You should wrap your legs around him, as this allows him to penetrate you more deeply and you're going to need to hold on tightly to each other. Now you both rock together, keeping your pelvises tight against each other, avoiding thrusting movements: there's no in and out action with this one. The idea is to rock gently to a climax. Women have 50 percent more chance of climaxing in this position, and the nonthrusting aspect of it makes him less likely to come. It's also a good position for coming at the same time.

Dr. David Delvin and Christine Webber, in *The Big O*, claim to have invented the aptly named PUSSY (Penis Underneath Scientifically Situated Yoni) position. This is simply an upside-down variation of the CAT. This time he gets to lie flat and you lower yourself onto the first part of his penis only. Your hips and chin should be below his and you'll bend his penis so that it stimulates your clitoris once again. You should aim for clitoral/penis contact and once again grind away. When doing this one take care not to bend his penis too far the wrong way!

If you and your partner have mismatched sex drives, turn to IDEA 8, *Starter's orders*.

Try another idea...

Don't forget that you can also improve clitoral stimulation by using lots of lube, moving more, and using longer stokes, and also by finding better ways to position yourself. For instance, use props like a chair, specially designed wedges, or a sling, all of which assist in getting the optimum angle. If you take a look at the two dozen *Kama Sutra* positions, you'll see that by simply moving the position of your pelvis or legs you can find a huge variety of positions without too much difficulty. Your legs can be straight, higher, curled on his chest, or he can lean forward and you can both squeeze with your thighs to produce the pressing position.

You might find it helpful to buy a book or DVD that depicts unusual and interesting sexual positions to try out. The DVD that accompanies the Femi-X herbal product contains a fifteen-minute presentation of twenty-seven sex positions designed to specially stimulate women based on the research of Dr. Lasse Hessel, the first to use ultrasound to study what actually happens inside the vagina during intercourse.

"Considerable variety is available to you through the simple expediency of changing the position of your legs."
MARVIN GROSSWIRTH, writer

Defining idea...

Experiment and see what new delights you can come up with!

How did it go?

Q **My partner and I are both overweight. What positions are good for us?**

A *There's an excellent article called "Fat Sex" on www.sexuality.org. The author (under the pseudonym of Dr. Katzenklutter) assures us that, in fact, obese people have few problems with their libido and can be extremely sexually active. His advice includes this: "If she has a big tummy, she can lift it away from her pubic region with both hands, at least until the man gets himself positioned between her thighs. If penetration is difficult, it can help to put one or more pillows under her buttocks." It can be easier for the heavier person to lie prone, but it's not problematic as long as they are prepared to take more of their weight on their knees. He also recommends that a woman on top with a large tummy can try facing back to front so that her abdomen does not come in contact with his.*

Q **It turns me off to think of fumbling around in different positions . . . Where do I go from here?**

A *A lot of people feel intimidated when they see classic poses like the Splitting of Bamboo from the Kama Sutra, but in reality, making small changes in the way you rest just one part of your body can make a huge difference in the way sex feels. Rather than thinking conceptually in terms of positions, just go on gut instinct and move around a little. If something feels good, then go for it!*

13

Toys R no fuss

**Better orgasms mean more effort, and a buzzing vibrator
and a drawer full of sex toys help you go at it longer. Will
you go on till the end?**

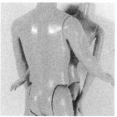

Using vibrators is the same as using your
hands, except that they're faster and never get
tired. You can use them all over your body or
dive in and cut to the chase.

Sex toys are great tools for experimenting with and are ideal for lazy days when you
need a helping hand. There's a mind-boggling range: vibrators, dildos, specific toys
for the anus and G-spot, clitoral and vulva massagers, as well as novelty and
waterproof versions. And a lot of us have them stuffed in our sock drawer, as
according to Durex's 2005 Global Sex Survey, more than half of couples use some
form of sex aid to spice up their sex life. Don't worry about introducing them into
sex games, you can do a lot more with them than just masturbation! Often men
enjoy the tickle of a vibrator against their penis or testicles and you can use
massagers and vibrators to stimulate each other's erogenous zones into action.

Some vibrators and dildos tend to be cheaper, more traditional models that look
like a fake penis, but the trend is to use better quality materials like silicone and

Here's an idea for you...

Masturbate with more than one sex toy. You can use a dildo/vibrator in your vagina and combine this with a vibrator tickling your clitoris (or Vielle's finger gloves). If you really want to push the boundaries, you can use an anal plug as well. You stand more chance of having better orgasms if you have more than one area being stimulated.

Pyrex glass and to incorporate new technology into the designs. The best thing about this, according to Cathy Winks, author of *The G-Spot*, is that "Manufacturers are now producing insertable vibrators and dildos that are curved to match the natural shape of the vagina and rectum." Some men might feel intimidated by a huge dong-shaped dildo, but they're less likely to be threatened by products which don't even look like a sex aid. The Fresh Vibes from www.funfactory.de have an animal design incorporated into their length. In an interview, spokesperson Jill-Evelyn Hellwig explained: "Many of our customers are women with children and they need something that's not going to be problematic if their children come across it."

I visited this innovative German company that exports women-friendly toys all over the world. Their biggest market is Belgium where, statistically, every other woman has a Fun Factory product. Jill-Evelyn Hellwig said, "If someone has never bought a vibrator before, they'll stick with something simple. And then they realize that they're doing something for themselves and there's so much more that they can do and eventually they'll start this learning process." You do need to experiment to find out what materials and shapes appeal to you. If you don't feel comfortable about self-insertion, try a clitoral massager like the Fun Factory Layaspot, which simply sits over your pubic bone and hums away; it has different speeds and programs to vary the tempo. You can also keep it in place while you have sex with your partner (he'll share a bit of the thrill, too).

For details on anal play using sex toys turn to IDEA 14, Alternative erogenous zones.

Try another idea...

The first time you insert a sex toy, don't feel pressured to put it all in. You're more sensitive on the outer third of your vagina, so some women like to just nudge and stimulate this area. If your partner is using a toy on you, he can start by performing cunnilingus and then inserting a finger or two until you're ready, but always go slow and insert just a little. The time for shoving it in is when you're screaming with pleasure!

Specially curved toys also make it easier to find your G-spot. It's easier to turn off your vibrator, or use a dildo to find it first (generally the other end will be designed to tickle your clitoris to give you double stimulation). G-toys are the most problematic to fit, as the length of women's vaginas varies. There are a lot of toys out there and you need to experiment to find out what works for you. Really, every woman should have lots of different sex toys for different reasons, so start adding these to your Christmas list and build your own personal collection!

"The vibrator provides the strongest, most intense stimulation ever known. Indeed, it has been said that the electric vibrator represents the only significant advance in sexual technique since the days of Pompeii."
DR. HELEN SINGER KAPLAN, sex therapist

Defining idea...

How did
it go?

Q   Is there any danger in using sex toys?

A   *No, providing you use them in accordance with the manufacturer's
     instructions. For instance, vibrators that plug into the outlet must be kept
     away from water; some toys like "egg" vibrators and Silver Bullets are non-
     insertable. It's also important to clean them just with mild soap and water
     (disinfectant sprays can damage the vaginal floor). It's best to keep them in
     a dedicated glass or metal cabinet where they'll be dust-free and have a
     chance to air. Moderation is also recommended. According to the British
     tabloids, one Welsh woman had a mishap wearing vibrating underwear. She
     apparently fainted from the effects of her orgasm at a local supermarket.
     When the ambulance crew arrived her pants were still buzzing! I'll leave this
     to you to decide if this is a good or bad thing!*

**Q   My partner gets really wild when we use sex toys. How can I give
     him a taste of his own medicine?**

A   *He can be penetrated anally or orally with butt plugs or any flared
     vibrator/dildo. Use plenty of lube and take it slow. To take it a step further,
     you can use a strap-on harness; some of those sold in sex shops are for
     heterosexual couples. Be gentle and use lots of lube, experiment with dildo
     size, but note that the harness takes half an inch off the dildo's length.*

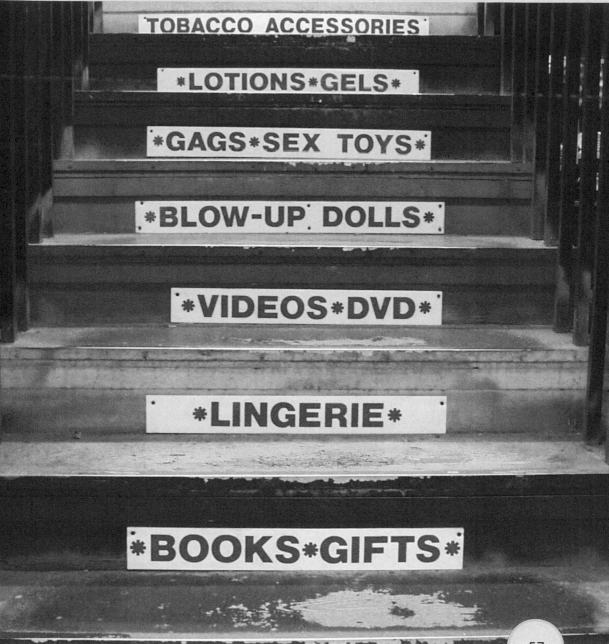

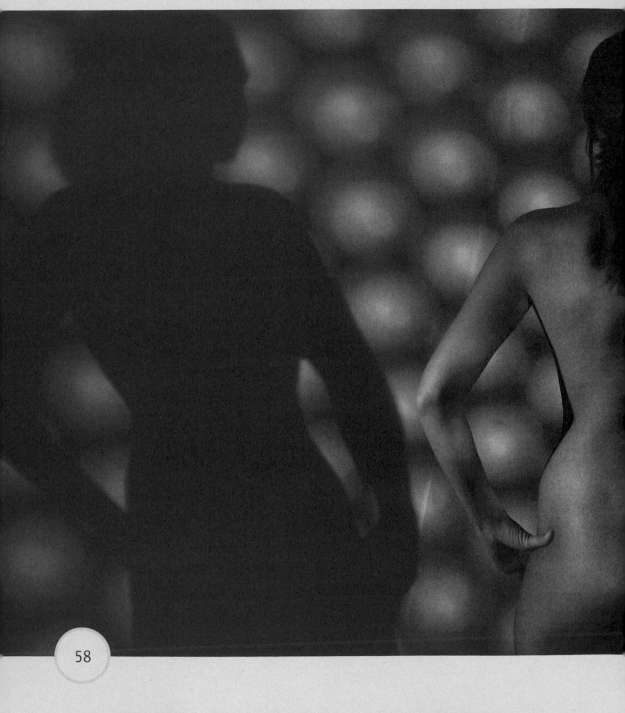

14

Alternative erogenous zones

All that glitters is not gold; the most obvious places may not be your top erogenous zones. Do you know what really turns you on?

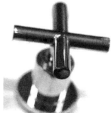

In a long-term relationship it's useful to continue finding new areas to make meaningful to your lover, and anal play is something you could both potentially enjoy.

The notion of us possessing "erogenous zones" was coined by a psychologist in response to 1920s fashion that revealed ladies' legs; J. C. Flugel suggested that sexually charged areas of the body fall in and out of fashion to keep our sexual curiosity on its toes. And almost any part of the body has the potential to be an erogenous zone: good lovers make use of the lips, neck, ears, scalp, shoulders, knees, and feet, *as well as* the obvious.

It's a good idea to extend your foreplay into making a sensory map of your lover's body to find out what makes him tick. Often we don't know what turns us on, so use foreplay as an opportunity to find out which buttons to press. Don't be surprised at what you find: Jonathan Margolis reports in *O: The Intimate History of the*

Here's an idea for you...

Place a vibrator or a plastic watch strap along your vagina and anus. Move it up and down and allow yourself to react to it. Does your anal area feel good when it's touched? What about the perineum, the bit in the middle? And which is best, your vagina or your clitoris?

Orgasm, "Large numbers of men and women are capable of achieving orgasm purely through earlobe manipulation—especially through mouth, tongue, and teeth." Writer Mik Scarlet, who is disabled, has written about how his nose became an erogenous zone.

We also respond to fashion. Writer Linda Dyett says that women's fashion plays on our secondary sexual characteristics, and most recently the midriff has become eroticized through women wearing short tops. If we're encouraged to dress to show off a particular part of the body, it's not surprising if we begin to feel sexier when it's touched.

Another theory is that a change in porn film practice has made activities like oral and anal sex more commonplace. The anal area can be highly erotic for both men and women, so it's worth experimenting.

If you'd like to try anal play, get your partner to give you really good foreplay first and get you warmed up. It's best to test the perineum first; if this feels nice being massaged, then you'll probably want some anal touch, too. Get your partner to use lots of lubricant (and maybe a glove if that makes you feel more comfortable) and to just use a finger to gently probe the area. You can also lick it (known as rimming);

use of dental dams over the area is optional. Some couples make anal play an extra feature of cunnilingus and gently tease just the outside of the anus.

To help find potential hot spots, spend more time indulging in foreplay—see IDEA 5, *Slippery when wet*.

Try another idea...

For full penetration, start with a finger or small butt plug first. Use lots of lube and take it slow. At first it may feel strange, but after the initial opening, it quickly becomes accommodating and pleasurable. You can use butt plugs with regular vaginal sex to get used to the feeling.

For full anal penetrative sex, forget what you see on porn videos. Use lots of lube (the anus has no natural lubrication) and use special condoms designed for anal sex. The most difficult part is initially getting the penis in there. It's best if you find a position where you can control entry with your hands (get him to push gently) so that he enters you at the right angle in some kind of comfort zone. It's easier for you to be in the position for missionary-style sex or for you to be on top to achieve this. When it's comfortable, he can increase the pace. Don't forget to add lube as you go along and stop if it starts to hurt. In the throes of passion, you might not notice any discomfort so remember it's how you feel *afterward* that's the real indicator of any soreness factor. Many women find it easier to come through anal penetration when they are on top because it stimulates the clitoris. It's also a different type of orgasm, so play around a little and find your next big thing.

"There is no part of the human body which is not sufficiently sensitive to effect erotic arousal and even orgasm for at least some individual in the populace."
DR. ALFRED KINSEY

Defining idea...

Q   Is anal sex damaging to your health?

A   *Yes and no. Porn stars who regularly do double anal penetration sometimes need stitches/surgery to repair their torn rectums. It's also possible to suffer from rectal incontinence. On the other hand, a penis or sex toy shouldn't be too problematic, as long as you monitor your comfort level. As Patrick Califia says in* Sensuous Magic: *"There's no reason why anal sex should be painful or traumatic. Most of us carry a lot of tension in our lower bodies, and the sensitive and vulnerable anus is the focal point for much of this stress. Pleasuring someone's butt can release years of pressure and discomfort." See www.puckerup.com for anal advice. Avoid touching the vaginal area with anything—fingers, penis—that has been in your anus as this can spread bacteria. Should you cut any part of your anus, get an anal cream or seek medical treatment right away. If your vagina feels a bit sore, you don't have to have sex, but, unfortunately, if your anus feels sore you'll still need to go to the toilet, so don't let it get to the stage where it hurts every time you have a bowel movement.*

Q   I tried anal sex but it was too painful. What can I do?

A   *Try anal* play *first and progress as far as you are able,* slowly. *Maybe a finger is enough for you. Just enjoy it.*

15

The great and the good

Alternative girl's-gotta-have-it zones within the vagina and that mysterious little thing, the G-spot. Talk about the best of both worlds!

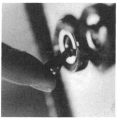

As well as the clitoris there are a number of hot spots that some women like stimulated. If this isn't your cup of tea, simply experiment and find out what tickles your fancy.

Don't dismiss the G-spot as just the latest fad. Dr. Gräfenburg "discovered" it in 1950, and it was popularized in the '80s, but we've known about it for a very long time. In 5 BC Galen wrote about the "female prostate," Chinese Taoist texts enthused about the "black pearl," and Indian Tantric texts revered the "sacred spot." So the G-spot has a long and honorable history.

For most women, the clitoris is their primary site of sexual pleasure. Unfortunately, because Freud criticized clitoral orgasms as being "immature," it's taken the best part of a hundred years for the clitoris as the prime female sex site to be acknowledged in recent times. Many researchers have been reluctant to go back to investigating vaginal orgasm, and only a small sample of women have taken part in

Here's an idea for you...

If you're having problems finding your G-spot, try searching for it after you've had one or more orgasms. The urethral sponge will have swelled, making it easier and more pleasurable to find.

trials. It's also more difficult to test for G-spot sensitivity, as some women need a lot of pressure to really feel it. Think of it as an added bonus.

The next time you take a shower do an internal examination. About three inches inside the vagina you're likely to find a spongy spot about the shape of an almond. If you can't locate it, try peeing, and you should be able to feel the urine moving through the vaginal wall. Remember, it's not *on* the wall; probe and feel for it *through* the wall. Em and Lo in *The Big Bang* describe it as a "kind of ceiling pipe surrounded by erectile tissue called the urethral sponge, sort of like insulation." For some people it's sensitive to the touch, but bear in mind that it can be quite hard to locate it yourself with a finger. Try using one of the special curved G-spot dildos like the Magic Wand, or better still, ask your partner to help you. Some women wait until they've already had an orgasm to probe the area. Some swear the best position is lying on their backs with their legs in the air, others lie on their side or kneel. Sex is very individual, so have a feel—is this a potential hot spot for you?

Defining idea...

"Over time I really 'came' to appreciate the delights that my G-spot had to offer."
ANNIE SPRINKLE, sex guru

You can add another dimension to your love life by opting to stimulate it more. When you masturbate, go for both clitoral and vaginal stimulation, using a finger or special curved dildo to touch the spot. If someone is going down on you, get them to insert a finger and touch you inside as well. Hitting both spots should produce deeper, more intense contractions. For penetration, you might want to experiment with positions that work the G-spot more, such as woman on top and rear entry. Or take a leaf out of the *Kama Sutra*: in the Raised Feet posture the woman lies on her back and lifts her knees while her partner kneels around her thighs and enters her.

Researchers have discovered that women with strengthened pelvic muscles are more likely to ejaculate. See IDEA 18, *Sexercise*, for special fitness tips.

Try another idea...

Some women are so stimulated by touching the spot, they ejaculate a clear fluid—don't worry, this is not urine. In *The G-Spot* Cathy Winks reported that the majority of her survey respondents who enjoyed G-spot stimulation also ejaculated. Just enjoy it if you can get it!

Other hot spots include the U-spot (the sensitive opening to the urethra), the X-spot on the cervix, and what the sex therapist Barbara Keesling calls "tenting"—the area behind the cervix which lifts up during sex to allow penetration of the space behind. Finally, find out if your G-spot is sensitive before having a hysterectomy—if it is, you can have a supra-cervical operation where they leave the cervix in. You don't want to find out too late!

"The function of the 'prostate' is to generate a juice which makes women more libidinous with its pungency and saltiness and lubricates their sexual parts in agreeable fashion during coitus . . . Here too it should be noted that the discharge from the female 'prostate' causes as much pleasure as does that from the male 'prostate.'"
REGNIER DE GRAAF, anatomist

Defining idea...

How did it go?

Q **I don't like the idea of female ejaculation. Isn't it unnatural for women to do this?**

A *Both sexes start off with the same basic material in the womb; it's only after six weeks that extra testosterone changes male sex organs into a penis form. Every structure in a man's sex organs is mirrored in a woman's, so it's not too surprising if women have the ability to ejaculate. Actually, scientists are still arguing over whether this is conclusive; only a small number of women have been tested to date. Obviously it's difficult to tell whether moisture comes from regular lubrication fluids or a spurt of ejaculate. Not every woman can do this, though some do claim to be able to (check out Sarah-Jane Hamilton's "gushing" porn tapes for proof). Don't feel embarrassed if you do spurt, it's a terrific compliment to your partner—it shows they are doing something right. As always with sex, keep a towel handy for any spillages.*

Q **The idea of having to hunt for yet another supposed hot spot gets me down. If I had sensitivity there, wouldn't I have found it by now?**

A *Examining yourself for potential pleasure zones shouldn't feel too much like hard work once you start to reap the benefits. Make a mental note to look into this on a rainy day and let your curiosity get the better of you. It could be that you are not especially sensitive in this area, but bear in mind that all of your muscles in the pelvic floor area are interconnected, so it's difficult—especially in the heat of passion—to figure out what feels best where.*

16

Extra credit

Once you've gotten there, perhaps you won't want to come back down. For multiple orgasms or extra stimulation, lend yourself a hand.

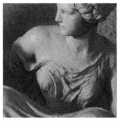

If you're having problems with orgasms, skip this section: but if you are hungry for more, here are some simple techniques to make you insatiable.

In the ancient world women were seen as being naturally more rampant than men. In Greek myth a man called Tiresias spent seven years as a woman and was then asked by Zeus which experience was best. When he said that women enjoy sex more than men, the gods blinded him for giving the "wrong" answer. Dr. Mary Jane Sherfey, the psychiatrist and author, concluded that one orgasm was not enough to satisfy the average female; three to five would be satisfactory, indeed, if time permitted: "Theoretically, a woman could go on having orgasms indefinitely, if physical exhaustion did not intervene." Wow!

Women are more multiorgasmic than men because they don't have to go through what's called the refractory period for so long. Masters and Johnson identified four stages of arousal: excitement, plateau, orgasm, and resolution. We all have to go

Here's an idea for you...

Give your man three to four minutes to cool down after you've had sex, then roll on top of him and manipulate yourself on his softened penis. If it's floppy, you'll be able to roll around on it, stimulating your clitoris better. You'll be surprised at how good it feels—and he might want to come again, too!

through each stage to get to the next one. Ironically, women who have problems having orgasms get stuck at the plateau stage, while multiorgasmic women revel in it; we're already there after we've come so it's relatively easy to build up to another.

There are two types of multiple orgasms. Sequential multiples come close together (two to ten minutes apart); the classic way is for a woman to come through oral sex and then to follow this with another during penetrative sex. A wilder ride is serial multiple orgasms that come right after each other like a roller-coaster ride. This occurs when all the hot spots are being stimulated (preferably more than two at once) and the best position is woman on top because you have more control. Of course, you should also be prepared to lend yourself a hand and to stimulate your clitoris/anus or alternative erogenous zone with your hand or vibrator.

The first step to getting there is to believe it will happen. Watch a video that features this if you're not convinced. Allowing yourself more time is also crucial. Dr. David Delvin and Christine Webber in *The Big O* say, "One of the curses of modern life is that women do not allow themselves enough time for sex—and for orgasms." They suggest allowing at least two hours for an extra-hot session.

You could start by practicing first with masturbation. If you feel too sensitive immediately after orgasm, wait for a minute and resume the action. If necessary, start to work on another area: clitoris, G-spot, breasts, the outer vaginal lips, or anus—you're trying to get the sensations to overlap with each other to mount up again. Once you've perfected this, play with your partner. Most men are motivated to please their women as many times as possible!

It's easy to climax again if you work more than one hot spot, so take a look at IDEA 14, *Alternative erogenous zones*, to cover all bases.

Try another idea...

Another technique, "peaking," plays with your arousal level. This is something men have more experience with (if you're using a condom maybe he waits for you to come first before succumbing to temptation). In a *Psychology Today* article—"Beyond Orgasmatron"—Barbara Keesling says, "As you make love, note your arousal levels on a scale from one to ten, with ten being orgasm. As you reach each level, briefly stop and allow your arousal to subside so that, rather than shooting for the moon, your arousal rides in a wave-like pattern." You can also fool your body into coming with another technique—"plateauing"—where you mimic some of the physical aspects of orgasm by squeezing your PC muscles, speeding up your breathing, and tensing your arm or leg muscles. Keesling claims you can train your body into responding to climax effortlessly at will. It's really a question of keeping going, experimenting, and devoting far more time to enjoying all of your pleasure zones!

"Sex is like money; only too much is enough."
JOHN UPDIKE

Defining idea...

How did it go?

Q Are women's orgasms different than men's? My boyfriend has had enough after just one!

A   *Yes. As well as having more potential to be multiorgasmic, women experience orgasms over a wider area. Jonathan Margolis in* O: The Intimate History of the Orgasm *says, "The biggest difference is, rather, that orgasmic feelings in men are localized in the immediate genital area of penis and testicles, while for women orgasmic sensations are felt throughout the pelvic area." This involves involuntary contractions of the vaginal walls, uterus, and rectal sphincter because our PC muscles are all interlinked, in an area generally known as the "orgasmic crescent." Of course, you can experience different types of orgasms; possible types include vaginal, clitoral, nipple, dream, and G-spot ones. The list is probably endless!*

Q Why do women have the capacity for more intense and multiple orgasms?

A   *Some anthropologists believe that evolutionary forces have made the clitoris the "mate meter"—a selective mechanism for choosing more loving and compassionate partners. In* What's Love Got to Do with It? *anthropologist Meredith Small suggests menstruation is a "biological defense" to keep bacteria from sperm out of our reproductive tracts and that the female capacity for multiple orgasms is designed to regulate the movement of sperm to improve reproductive success. It seems that if we have multiple partners we have the ability to choose the sperm of our mates; if we have an affair we are twice as likely to get impregnated by our lovers.*

17

Giving it some

It feels good to give pleasure to your partner. You want to hear those moans. Here's how to drive your man wild—put a few tricks up your sleeve.

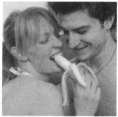

Knowing you are a good lover gives you confidence, and making him see stars is an incentive for him to make an extra special effort to get you off!

Men find it easier to have an orgasm than women, but because their goal is ejaculation they often miss out on getting their full quota of sensual pleasure. In their *Illustrated Guide to Extended Massive Orgasm* Steve and Vera Bodansky reckon that "They miss probably 80 percent of each stroke," so encourage him to slow down. Take a more active role so that he can take a backseat and enjoy himself more.

Just kissing him is sexier if you play with his lower lip. Suck it into your mouth and run your tongue down to his chin, it should send a shock wave he'll feel in his penis. The neck is also a known erogenous zone, particularly the area under the Adam's apple. Men also respond well to massage, but before you get down to it search for other hot spots. Does he like having his nipples touched? Use your hands, tongue, and a hot mouth to give him the once-over.

Here's an idea for you...

Don't just mount him, do a reverse girl-on-top position so he can get a good look at you. Just before he climaxes, reach for his ankles and feel for his pressure points just below his ankle bones and press them as he comes. It'll feel electric!

Don't forget to talk dirty to him, and let him see as much of your body as possible. Men are much more receptive to sight and smell, so if you want to give him a handjob, do it so he can see your excited vagina. It's less work if you use lubricant on your hands—his penis will automatically bump up and down, so use pressure that feels good for him. The most sensitive part of the penis is the frenulum (where the head meets the shaft) so stimulate this extra well. One technique is to keep one hand on the penis at all times stroking its head (preferably slick with lube) while your other hand gives long strokes to the rest of his penis. You can add twists, move both hands differently, or use one hand to nudge his perineum. Men like to have their testicles played with, and any time you stimulate multiple areas it boosts his arousal.

Men love oral sex. To increase his pleasure, tie your hair back so he can see you doing it; even better, do it on your knees so that he can cop an eyeful of your breasts, and extended neck. Brush your lips against his head, tickle him with your tongue, and vary the sucking strokes. Some men like to masturbate the penis with their hand while you suck the top; encourage him to do whatever feels good. If you're confident with fellatio, you could try to deep throat him. To do this you need to be able to control your gag reflex, which is easier to do with your neck straight. If you're not sure what to do, get him to move your head in the right rhythm.

During sex, just as he should be looking to stimulate your clitoris, look for his hot spots. Kneading the testicles works well, particularly the seam of it which contains lots of nerve endings. Some men can orgasm just from prostate stimulation, the male G-spot, which is just inside the anus. You could probe this with a finger or insert a well-greased butt-plug, but check first if he's game. Prostate orgasms feel different and are more of a full body experience, so stimulating this can give him a completely new feeling. The ultimate in female power is to use a strap-on on him. In *Brief Encounters* Emily Dubberley says, "About 30 percent of strap-ons sold by sex shops go to straight couples," so it's not uncommon. Use lots of lubricant and go slowly. It could be that he only wants to take part of it, or even just experience the psychological thrill of your "penis" tickling his nether regions.

Experiment with what works for both of you. Relax and slow down; his orgasm is better if it is delayed, so tease him and take him to the brink a few times. He'll appreciate the difference!

Most men love anal play, although they might not ask for it. Check out IDEA 14, *Alternative erogenous zones*, for tips.

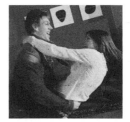

"Remember that in the beginning: An erection is like a dog with a concussion; it's just as likely to roll over and play dead as it is to come when you call."
SHARYN WOLF, couples therapist

How did
it go?

Q   Why should I play with his anal area? Isn't that odd?

A   *Both men and women are receptive to anal stimulation, so a man isn't "odd"
just because he likes being touched down there. Some men can distinguish
between regular orgasms and those triggered by prostate stimulation. The
difference in sensation is because the prostate connects to the pelvic nerve
pathway. If he's receptive, he's opening himself up to a whole new
orgasmic potential initiated by you, so he should be pretty happy about it!*

Q   Why are men so hung up on coming?

A   *They experience orgasm differently than a woman. Once it starts, it can't be
stopped because it's involuntary, although some say orgasm and ejaculation
are not the same thing. Jonathan Margolis, in* O: The Intimate History of the
Orgasm, *says, "A controversial (and lately fashionable) body of opinion
exists that orgasm and ejaculation in men are quite separate functions; that
physiologically, ejaculation is simply a reflex that occurs at the base of the
spine, an involuntary muscle spasm resulting in the ejection of semen and
felt only in the penis, whereas orgasm is somehow much more than that, an
unspecified 'whole body experience' produced by clenching muscles
throughout the body to avoid the penis being sensitized." Watch this space!*

18

Sexercise

It's not just your butt that you need to tone up. Simple fitness tips to pep up your stamina and get you ready for the long haul.

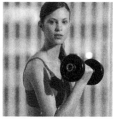

Strengthening your PC muscles increases arousal rate, sensations, and stamina. The technique has also inspired a range of fun toys such as the vaginal barbell—a much more exciting form of home gym!

Any exercise is good for you, but the optimum way to achieve better orgasms is to strengthen and tighten your pelvic floor—the actual muscles that do the most work during sex. This is the group of six muscles that control and hold in place all of the holes in that area: the urethra, vagina, and anus. In modern life we sit rather than squat, so often these muscles are weakened. Regular "love squeezes" tighten and tone the muscles, a surefire way to put the zip back into your love life!

Here's an idea for you... **Get your partner to help you do your Kegels. He should insert two fingers into your vagina and then open up his fingers inside while you try to close them with your vaginal sphincter muscles. You can do this ten times and incorporate it as part of your foreplay.**

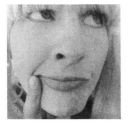

This is not a new idea. As far back as 800 BC, Chinese texts praised the virtues of a woman having a firm grip, and in Ancient Japan *Ben Wa* balls, which give the wearer pleasurable sensations, were invented by an unknown courtesan—they also improve the grip of the PC muscles. We've all seen the videos where accomplished strippers can shoot darts and ping-pong balls from their strong, trained vaginas. Not that I'm suggesting you work to this intensity!

You've probably heard of Kegel exercises. They were designed to offset the problems of urinary incontinence, especially in pregnant women, but the bonus side effect is a tightened, toned vagina. Dr. Joshua Davies first suggested using the exercises, but it was Dr. Arnold Kegel who popularized them. He never intended them to be performed alone though; they were carried out in his office with his Kegel Perineometer. Nowadays, people are encouraged to do this at home, although it's tricky at first to find the right muscles.

The best way to find your PCs is to put a finger in your vagina and clench your muscles. You should be able to feel pressure on your finger. Very often, people use the wrong muscles, so have a few goes until you feel something. Try more fingers or a dildo if you're having difficulty. Once you've found your muscles, clench them, and try to clench your anus, vagina, and urethra muscles separately. Clench and release. Try to do ten contractions, take a rest, and go for ten more. Breathe evenly throughout. When you've got the hang of it, try to do them every day or as often as you can manage.

For more tips about understanding your vagina, check out IDEA 3, *Sticky fingers*. This encourages you to learn about the hormonal processes that go on each month.

Try another idea...

About a third of all women have weak pelvic floors, so that means a lot of us have room for improvement. Dr. Kegel suggests you need to squeeze your PC muscles 30–100 times per day, but in *The 7 Minute Sex Secret* fitness expert Martica Heaner says that to enhance your sex life this is not enough: "You need to train for sex. You must practice the exercises in such a way that they replicate the rhythms, body positions, and forces present during sex." She suggests you need to squeeze harder or longer or use some type of resistance like vaginal barbells. We have two types of muscles—slow and fast twitch—and we need to exercise both

"In popular literature, Kegel's exercises are most frequently described as those which have to do with the 'stopping and starting the flow of urine.' As a simple means of pubococcygeus muscle identification, this test is educational—but only for those who already have strong muscles. It was never intended to be the 'instructional tool' that it has become in women's magazines."
JOHN PERRY AND LESLIE TALCOTT HULLETT, incontinence specialists

Defining idea...

Defining idea…

"Many women spend hours toning their bodies, but focus most on the outside and forget about the muscles inside."
MARTICA K. HEANER, writer

types to get results. This is why you should alternate between power squeezes and quick flutters. It's been proven that using some form of resistance (a dildo or vaginal barbell) gets results three times faster. The vaginal barbell is a special kind of dildo especially for PC exercises, although you can substitute a regular dildo if you prefer. Dr. Dodson's Exercise Wand is made from stainless steel and will change angle when you contract the pelvic muscles so you know you are doing them correctly. Similarly, the Vielle Pelvic Floor Toning System has a patented locator to ensure correct positioning, and an indicator to ensure you use the right muscles. An alternative is the Vaginal Exercise Egg. At first practice with it lying down, but when your muscles are stronger you can walk around with it. Advanced users can tie weights to the string for greater resistance training. You should alternate between fast, slow, and weighted clenches and even better, test out your clenching skills during sex with your partner's penis.

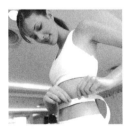

Q **I've tried doing Kegel exercises, but so far haven't seen any effect. How long should it take?** *How did it go?*

A *Dr. Kegel got his patients to practice these exercises two to three times a day for up to an hour, but remember these were people suffering from an incontinence problem, rather than just needing to jazz up their sex life. Kegel did suggest that around forty hours of training is all that is needed. Martica Heaner suggests seven minutes a day; other sexperts suggest ten clenches on waking and ten when you go to bed. The good thing about Kegels is that you can do them at any time of the day—standing up, lying down, walking—so try to fit them in where you can. In general, it takes about six to twelve weeks to see a real difference.*

Q **My boyfriend is fascinated by my new "hobby." How can I put this to practical use in bed?**

A *Practicing your clenches during sex is an excellent way to carry out the exercises. Don't forget to release each contraction completely so he can feel the full effects. Martica Heaner suggests squeezing before he enters; the muscles at the opening of your vagina respond most to Kegel exercises.*

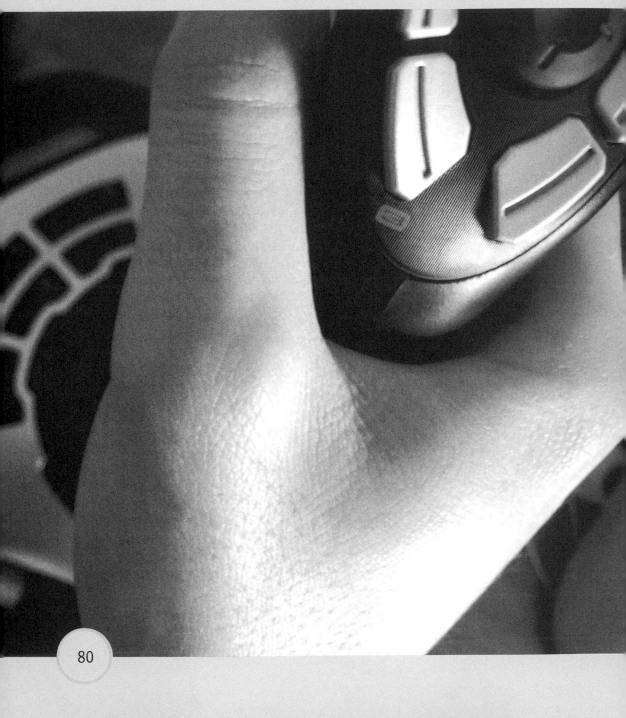

19

Tell it like it is

Point your lover in the right direction. Assert your sexual identity. Let the cat out of the bag and express yourself to lovers, in your diary, or under a nom de plume on the net.

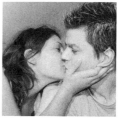

Once you know what you like, the next step is to signal this to your lover. Psychologists advise that communication is important, but there are many ways to make your desires known.

Talking is easy when things are going right. The problems start when things get jaded or go downhill. Often couples walk an emotional minefield during such a time, each afraid to let on to the other that something is amiss. Talking about the big "O" is particularly difficult because many people are afraid of hurting their partner's feelings. Good sex is regarded as a right, something that should come naturally, but like everything else in life, it takes a little effort. Sex therapist Aline P. Zoldbrod says in *Sex Talk* that one of the best ways to communicate about sex is to build on your positive experiences: "Flip through your memories and zero in on one time that really blew the others out of the water." Once you work out the red-hot bits that turn you both on, use these more often in your sexual repertoire. Don't shy away from talking about sexual dislikes, too: if you hate it, it's a bitch when he sticks his finger in your anus, putting you off just as you're about to come.

Here's an idea for you...

Ask your lover to tell you a story; it can be anything. But once you've established this, ask him to tell you about his first sexual experience, or the first time he had sex with you. Work up to him confessing his "fantasy" story with all the details he never normally reveals.

To get you in the mood for talking frankly, you could watch a film about sex (erotic or otherwise) to make the subject easier to discuss. If you can't bring yourself to watch anything erotic yet, talk about the married couple in *American Beauty* or any film that features modern relationships. You could also set aside a corner of your home as a den where you can snuggle and talk to each other. Alternatively, signal a special time—Sunday brunch, perhaps—for sexy conversation.

Zoldbrod suggests going to a bookstore and studying the sex books together (a turn-on, at least!). Another tip from her is to draw a "body" map signifying which areas you definitely like to be touched, which not, and which ones you are unsure about. If you don't feel you can sit and discuss this "cold," then ask to be blindfolded and simply cry out in pleasure to illustrate; use ice or a tongue dipped in hot tea to help get the message across—the skin is the biggest erogenous zone and temperature differences accentuate pleasure.

Defining idea...

"Women are never disarmed by compliments. Men always are. That is the difference between the sexes."
OSCAR WILDE

Some people don't bring up sex because they are afraid of sharing too much detail about their past. It's a myth that it's possible to have too few lovers, or too many. A good way to make this scenario more comfortable is to start by sharing funny things. For example, you could tell your partner something like, "You know the first time I ever used a tampon,

I inserted the whole thing, cardboard carton and all because I didn't know I had to push the tampon out." This opens the floodgates to trading secrets and revealing more. To get over the risk of sharing personal histories, Zoldbrod suggests telling "two hypotheticals and one truth," with your partner having to guess which one is true. You can choose to reveal the final truth when it feels comfortable.

To get you in the mood for intimacy, watch an inspirational film. See IDEA 50, Wet scenes, for movie suggestions.

Try another idea...

There are also emails, texting, phone calls, and journals. Some people find it easier to talk dirty over the phone because they can let their guard down without having to reveal their body language. Another tip is to write down your ideal fantasy and leave it somewhere your lover can read it. Make it sizzling hot, just how you'd like it to happen.

Some people reveal their darkest fantasies to strangers they meet anonymously in chat rooms. This can be addictive and time consuming. In one way this helps you to find out what you want, and is perfect for masturbation fans, but don't forget not everyone wants to actually live out their fantasy. It's better to consummate this in real life, so get on down and express yourself!

"Before you get into new sexual situations, you should always do yourself the favor of thinking about what you want out of them. Even if you are in a long-term relationship and just want things to change, you need to be able to understand for yourself and be able to tell your lover what those 'things' are."
ALINE P. ZOLDBROD

Defining idea...

83

How did
it go?

Q   Why should I get all analytical about sex?

A   *The way you communicate your hot spots is up to you. You can signal by
     screaming when your lover touches the right place or talking about it over
     dinner. It's important to get those sexual boundaries down pat because
     doing so improves your sex life. A survey of more than 100,000 married
     women showed that women who are more able to talk about their sex life
     had sex more often and were more orgasmic. If you are not in the habit of
     doing so already, then start right now.*

**Q   I've been with my partner for fifteen years so we have nothing new
     to say to each other; when we do talk it ends in an argument.
     What now?**

A   *Perhaps once you knew each other's most intimate thoughts, but it's
     possible that one or both of you have changed. Zoldbrod says, "Our bodies
     and our sex lives are renewable resources. Sensitivities and willingnesses
     change over time." This means we should be open to change and not be
     surprised if one of you has new ideas. As for arguing, this is a normal part
     of a relationship: at least you are communicating something you dislike mid-
     tantrum.*

20

Mind games

Not enough hours in the day? Too tired? The most erotic place is the mind, so role-play and snatch back time to salvage those precious moments.

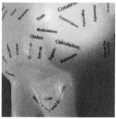

Building up an elaborate fantasy life is fun, creative, and free, plus you get to know more about the hidden depths of each other's psyche!

One of the advantages of being in a long-term relationship is that you get to know how the other person ticks. Even if you're not conscious of it, you've built up a system of codes, rituals, and associations that instantly signals your mood. For instance, if you're into playing with ice cubes during foreplay, a seemingly innocuous glass filled with ice takes on a whole different meaning. There's a lot of mileage to be gained from playing out your fantasies.

Decades ago, Alfred Kinsey showed that we actively fantasize during masturbation; women do this around 66 percent of the time and men nearly all the time. It goes without saying that being able to act out your favorite fantasy does wonders for

Here's an idea for you... **Remember your dolls' tea set and the fun you had with it? Get your partner to secretly set up lots of things in small dishes that you can use erotically such as ice, warm water, egg white (a natural lubricant), ice cream, honey, pieces of fruit, rose petals, sex toys. Your partner blindfolds you and gets you to investigate what's waiting inside each dish and helps you to make the most of it . . .**

your sex life. These are mind games that rely on trust, communication, and trying to serve someone else's needs: all good tools for building a healthy relationship. Common sexual fantasies that couples role-play involve power dynamics such as master and pupil, nurse and patient, and being taken against your will. This is no surprise given that women are encouraged to be desirable but passive—just take a look at the way lovers force themselves roughly on the heroines in romantic fiction! Kath Albury says in *Yes Means Yes*, "The popularity of the bodice-ripping, pseudo-rape fantasies springs from the good girl's very real and frustrating desire to have wild sex without being called a slut or sicko."

Other scenarios might be that you're a virgin or meeting for the first time: it's really your call.

To act out a fantasy, first of all you have to find out what turns you on and work out your boundaries. (If you want to walk all over him with high-heeled shoes, it could be he insists you throw a blanket over him first.) Perhaps you want to eroticize things you find not so good, like a Caesarean scar or needing to have safe sex. The delicious thing about head play is that you can talk over the details first at length and use this to get each other off. You might want to invest in some props to make it more authentic. For women, a wig and certain types of shoes and/or underwear are very effective, and it's a great excuse to play around with makeup, temporary tattoos, and accessories. Just like making a film, you come up with a script, work out the characters, sets, and costumes, and then set it up so it's ready to roll.

Some couples have fun keeping the details secret until the big day when they get to enact it. And the delicious time spent in anticipation and preparation is crucial: it's like pre-programming your brain to have a massive orgasm. When the moment of truth comes, ensure that you have a safe word (or if you are tied up, a marble you can drop) so that you're both aware when the other wants to stop and come out of their role. It should be an invigorating sexual experience, but even if you felt your partner's ten out of ten orgasm, it's still wise to deconstruct events and check that you're both OK to continue on another day.

Constructing an elaborate fantasy that you can both get into is ideal for taking a shortcut to getting in the mood: he plays a certain music track or says the magic word and—*boom*—you're horny! This works if you indulge in it occasionally, so don't be afraid to act out. You can be whoever you want to be!

If you want to keep your dirty thoughts all to yourself, turn to **IDEA 27, Indecent proposal.**

Try another idea...

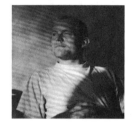

"Human beings have a fascinating capacity to connect any given meaning or feeling state with virtually any act."
PATRICK CALIFIA, author

Defining idea...

87

How did
it go?

Q Why should a "normal" person need fantasies anyway?

A *As Kinsey showed, fantasizing is a normal element of getting off. Some women actually need to fantasize while having sex with their partner in order to come. In Forbidden Flowers, Nancy Friday assures us, "If a sexual fantasy helps turn us on to a higher erotic pitch than we would ordinarily reach, it does not mean we are deficient lovers." Often things that are kinky for women are not categorized as such. A man who craves a high-heeled shoe has a fetish, but a desire for tall or black men is just seen as a preference. Kath Albury, author of Yes Means Yes, notes, "Even when women exhibit very clear fetishistic sexual tendencies, the 'f' word is so rarely used to describe them."*

Q My boyfriend has a fetish for me wearing rubber, which I don't understand, plus he gets jealous if I tell him too much about my fantasies. What should I do?

A *Most people who have a fetish have no motivation to change it because thinking about it is so pleasurable. As long as you're happy to go along with it, that's fine. You can always persuade him to modify it slightly or just keep his fantasies in his head. With his jealousy, my tip is not to make your fantasy elaborations too personal; for instance, don't tell him to pretend he's your ex-boyfriend, even if you still have a crush on him.*

21

Compromise positions

Quickie sex in half the time and ways to satisfy each other when you don't have time to go all the way.

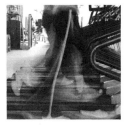

Like keeping up with regular exercise, good sex involves making a bit of a commitment, but here are some tips to put a little extra into those off days.

It's all very well waxing lyrical about leisurely techniques, but sometimes we just don't have time to put them into practice. A lot of us would rather catch up on shut-eye instead. The National Sleep Foundation polled 1500 adults in 2005 and found 58 percent are simply too tired for sex. And the less sex you have, the more this trend continues; sex-starved marriages are on the rise, and the latest acronym for modern couples is DINS (Double Income No Sex). Initiating sex when you're tired and don't feel like it can lead to less sleep, compounding the problem. Germaine Greer famously said, "No sex is better than bad sex," so if you're really beat go straight to sleep and postpone lovemaking until you're more alert.

Here's an idea for you...

If you don't feel like it right now, kiss your partner passionately and talk about the hot things you're going to do to each other next time you've got the opportunity for a long, passionate lovemaking session, and set the date!

However, sleepy lovers can improvise to speed things along. To get you warmed up, try starting foreplay earlier while you are watching TV and then you can finish off in the bedroom. If one of you showers at night, join them and have sex right there in the shower—one of the best positions for couples in a hurry is to do it standing up, and this way there's no need to clean up afterward. If he's not up to penetrating you, you can buy a dildo to stick on the shower wall for you to ride on and give him a full view.

Other tricks involve making use of new technology to get you aroused quicker. The Tantra Beam massager (tantrabeam.com) is an electric pulse device you wear on your wrist like a watch; the strap slips over your finger. You're still touching your partner with the feel of your own skin, but when you switch on the machine it literally electrifies your touch which makes for a quick thrill. (To really push the boundaries, he can wear this around his waist and turn his penis into a vibrator.) It's also good as a relaxing massager if you just want a bit of touchy-feely. In your regular lovemaking sessions, make a mental list of things that turn each other on and discover positions that make you come quicker for maximum effect (both men and women generally find it easier to come on top).

Defining idea...

"Nobody dies from lack of sex. It's lack of love we die from."
MARGARET ATWOOD

Also reinvent the quickie. Rather than thinking of it as compromise sex, keep such sessions extra special by restricting certain positions and predilections that you love just to these times.

To inject a little *oomph* into your fantasy life see IDEA 27, *Indecent proposal*.

Try another idea...

You don't need to fit a quick one in just before bed; you could ravish your partner ten minutes before you're due to meet friends when you're already dressed up, or take advantage of a quiet strip of sand at the beach. An optimal time for sex is first thing in the morning (men wake up with an erection) and if you're not feeling particularly fresh, keep a strip of chewing gum for instant invigoration by the bed. Have sex in the spooning position or doggy style if you don't want him to look at you too carefully without your makeup.

Making compromises is all about considering your partner. Try to make a bit of an effort to please each other. It could be that you allow yourself to be more enthusiastic about foreplay, or find other things to keep him interested, like giving him a striptease show while he masturbates, using sex toys on him, or talking dirty to get him off. Play around a little and find compromise solutions; if physically you're feeling unresponsive, there's no excuse to let your fantasy life flatline also. And getting a bit more active should give you the taste for more.

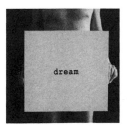

"A terrible thing happened to me last night again— nothing."
PHYLLIS DILLER

Defining idea...

How did it go?

Q   Why should I get involved in any kind of sexual activity?

A   *Humans crave touch, so even if you don't want to physically have intercourse, you can still hug your partner and find ways to get him off if he needs it. Sexual dissatisfaction is one of the biggest reasons for divorce, so don't avoid the issue if your partner has a different desire level. On the other hand, low-sex relationships are coming out of the closet—check out websites like Aven (www.asexuality.org) and The Frigadarium (which can be found at www.geocities.com/decussationofthepyramids) for info. Obviously, this is great if you both feel the same way, but a disaster if you don't. It's not just women who lose interest, either: Denise Donnelly of Georgia State University studied seventy-five married couples who were sexually inactive and in 60 percent of the cases it was the men who had stopped.*

Q   Do we really need sex?

A   *Not in the same way as food and sleep, but sex has lots of physical and psychological benefits. Arousal releases endorphins, which relieve anxiety and boost our immune system. Barbara Keesling says in* Beyond Orgasmatron, *"With all the mental and physical benefits of sex, it's like we're walking around with a complete health care system inside our own body."*

22

Seeing is believing

Are you doing the grown-up thing—looking at each other enough during sex? Here are some ways to position yourself so that you can see how you feel.

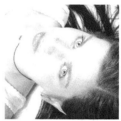

Doing something as simple as looking at each other properly during foreplay and sex can increase intimacy and give you "full-bodied" orgasms.

Literal "love making," with lots of eye contact and tenderness, heightens the connection between you and your partner. Of course, good sex comes in lots of varieties, but if you're not really emotionally attached to someone, you're less likely to look into their eyes. Sight is the dominant sense for most of us; as Tracey Cox says in *Superdate*: "Around 55 percent of us 'see the world,' 15 percent 'hear' it, and 30 percent 'feel' it." We're also the only primates that have developed virtually all our erogenous zones on the front of our bodies, so let's make use of our sight and enjoy the view.

You might want to start by looking at your partner more when he's naked. Chat to him when he's in the bath or shower. Can you appreciate his body visually when you're not feeling horny? Learn the little gestures, like the small hand and facial movements he makes, so that you can read his expressions.

Here's an idea for you... **Try making love in positions where you spend more time gazing into each other's eyes. The Inverted Embrace from the *Kama Sutra* is ideal. The woman is on top and lies prone against the man's chest, pressing her breasts to his body, then she moves her hands down to grip his hips. With your upper body flat down, you can rock to orgasm and exchange loving glances all the way.**

Once you have this intimacy, you'll know how to read him the next time you get flirty. Find out what things turn him on (does he like lacy undies, stockings, leather, a hair-free zone?) and get him to wear those things that please you. Perhaps he looks good in that tight T-shirt or wearing just a leather jockstrap. Being able to turn each other on visually is a shortcut to arousal. Then you can move on to sensual kissing. Look into each other's eyes and kiss deeply. You want to see the effect your passion has on your lover. If you do oral sex, choose positions so that you can see each other. If he licks you, pull your knees up so you can see his face, and get him to look up at you every so often. Likewise, pull your hair back so he can see you fellating him. Keep kissing each other on the lips every so often, and return to face and eye contact as your main position.

The missionary position is the classic one for keeping lip and eye contact, but there are other face-to-face positions that feel more personal. The Fitter-In from the *Kama Sutra* has both of you sitting facing each other with your legs over his hips. Grip each other's arms and rock in position and connect with your eyes. For even cozier variations, sit up in his lap (still facing each other) with your legs around his back. An alternative is to lie side-by-side in a gentle, relaxed position, your legs intertwined and holding hands. It's easier to control the thrust of penetration like this, too. All these positions allow you to cuddle, caress, and look lovingly into each other's eyes as well as have sex.

For a complete contrast, experiment with what happens when you cut off one of the senses in IDEA 37, *Eyes wide shut*.

Try another idea…

If you like to be on top, try sitting astride him while he's in a chair; it gives you more leverage and gravity works to make your thrusts feel deeper, and you can snuggle in comfort. If you're lying on top of him on a bed, try leaning backward a little and resting one hand on his knee to get a better look at your lover. Put a pillow under his head to give him a better view and experiment with eye contact and body position until you get the balance of lust and love right!

"The eye is the window of the human body through which it feels its way and enjoys the beauty of the world."
LEONARDO DA VINCI

Defining idea…

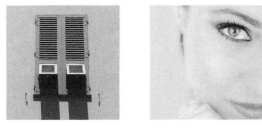

How did it go?

Q **Is it really sexy to see him brushing his teeth and stuff like that?**

A *It's intimate and whether it looks sexy or not will depend on how he looks and carries himself (and I hope he does look hot). It's good to be naked in front of each other. Photographer Petter Hegre took thousands of pictures of his first wife in the bath, getting dressed and so on, and captured the intimate nature of their relationship in the photo-book, My Wife. Feeling comfortable in your skin and being able to cuddle up and touch when you're naked, without any sexual stimulation, is kind of a prerequisite to an intimate relationship. Casanova (who knew a thing or two) used mirrors and candles to give his lovers plenty to feast their eyes on.*

Q **My boyfriend just isn't into looking at me when we have sex. Is it a guy thing?**

A *Maybe. Psychologist Bruce Dorval videotaped people talking to their same-sex friends; at all ages girls and women looked at each other directly, but boys and men sat at angles and only glanced at each other occasionally. Take the lead and kiss him ardently, keep returning to the base position of face-to-face kissing. Once you get him to open his eyes you can't go wrong!*

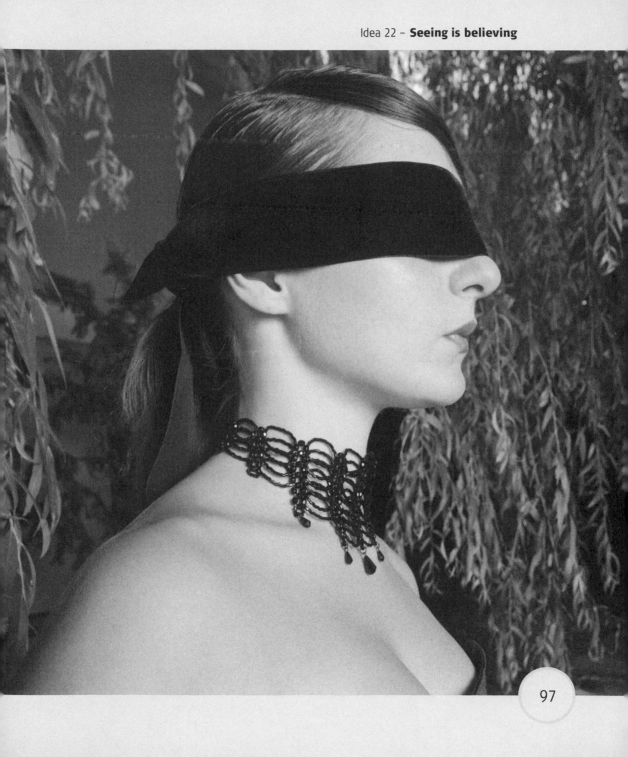

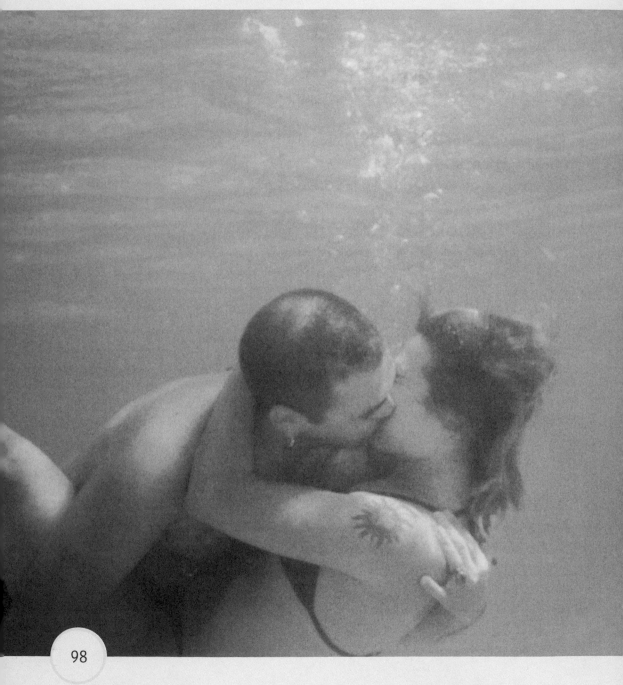

23

Sex in water

There's something exciting about a little splashing and thrashing around in water, especially if it's combined with a bit of aqua erotica!

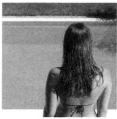

All your favorite sex toys come in waterproof versions, and the versatility of water makes it the ideal medium for adding the X factor to your sex life.

Water is the most essential element of life, so it's not surprising we feel revitalized when we're splashing around in it. Our bodies feel lighter immersed in it (the water takes some of the weight) and the sensation of water on our bodies kick-starts our blood circulation. In addition, during water play we're probably going to be scantily clad and doing some invigorating form of exercise. To top it off, hopefully our bodies will be being given a dose of vitamin D from the sun: all the raw ingredients for feeling raunchy and playful. It's not surprising that sex on a summer vacation seems the best we have all year.

Of course, it's not so easy to literally have sex in water. If you're lucky enough to have your own whirlpool or private swimming pool, this makes life easier, although you should keep a tube of silicone lube nearby as penetrative sex in water tends to wash

Here's an idea for you... **Play around with a sexy inflatable like the E-Z Rider Rocker and Dong available from Xandria.com. It's a bit like the hopper balls you played with as a kid, except this has a dildo that you can insert and ride on. It makes a great bath time accessory (use gently in a regular tub) and comes into its own for secluded swimming spots. When you've finished, simply deflate.**

away your natural moisture. Some women have said that after having sex in a swimming pool the chlorine has made them sore but using the lube should help, and, anyway, water is the perfect medium for productive play and massage. You can always finish up on dry land somewhere to take things further.

Pool accessories like floats, inflatable chairs, and toys are all great for horsing around with. Use the opportunity to throw yourself at each other and play games on inflatable shapes. If you're in a romantic mood, use floats to support your partner's head and/or lower torso. Get your partner to close his eyes and gently wade through the water until his body is completely relaxed. If you have privacy, you can move up to genital foreplay, or use an underwater clit massager like the Waterdancer toy. If you don't have these options, use the water to de-stress and warm each other up before you move on to dry land, and to the real thing. If you're on a secluded lake, there's also fun stuff like an inflatable trampoline that's great for bouncy, gyrating sex. It's best to wear a life jacket just in case, and you could even go for it while floating in life jackets. Water sports like snorkeling are great in themselves, so it's an extra bonus if your partner massages you erotically as you're swimming along. Again, take care of safety and incorporate floats if you're in deeper water. And remember that in most places genital fondling and sex in public is illegal!

These days, there are loads of waterproof sex toys that help you to get off discreetly. For instance, you could insert Fun Factory pleasure balls and then go for a swim in your local pool or sit in a spa. There's also the Wireless Waterproof Vibrating Panty with a wireless waterproof micro-orb that fits into the pants. Wear a swimsuit over it and nobody will notice.

If you get the opportunity, all those floating chairs and inflatables make for great oral sex locations. Turn to IDEA 7, *Get him to use his mouth*, for useful tips.

Try another idea…

Alternatively, there are plenty of bath and shower accessories that can be put to good use. Almost every type of sex toy imaginable comes in a waterproof version and you can get dildo accessories to stick on the shower door or side of the bath. Some toys look perfectly innocuous: for instance, there's a Sponge vibrator that gets you clean as well, and a Ducky vibrator that gets going when you give the little fellow a squeeze.

If you don't like the idea of sticking something inside you, the Layaspot clitoris massager from the Fun Factory is perfect for you. It's waterproof and has a range of vibrations and fits snugly over the pubic bone. Simply lie back and relax and let the machine do the work. Mmm . . .

*"If I were called in
To construct a religion
I should make use of water."*
PHILIP LARKIN

Defining idea…

How did
it go?

Q **I'd like to try masturbation in the bath but have problems getting turned on there. Any ideas?**

A   *Yes. If dirty stories give you a helping hand, there are two possibilities. You could try listening to erotic audio CDs like the Herotica series, or Aqua Erotic publishes sexy stories (appropriately around the theme of water) and these are cleverly designed in a plastic-backed book that is completely waterproof. (Apparently, readers have tested it with a range of other fluids, too.) If you have a partner to help you, get him to try doing stuff like washing your hair, which is amazingly sexual but is an underrated erotic activity in the West.*

Q **We want to try having sex in water but need to practice safe sex. Is it possible to do this?**

A   *The jury's out on that one. Condoms weren't really designed to be used underwater, so there's no real data to establish reliability. I suggest that you use the shower as an alternative, or get your partner to use a clitoral massager or waterproof sex toy on you underwater. You'll probably find that titillating enough to meet your fantasies. If you do decide to go ahead using condoms, then it's better to use polyurethane ones rather than latex, or try the female condom and use it with a silicone lube like Eros. Happy splashing!*

24

Dangerous liaisons

There's nothing like a little attention to make someone feel sexy. Flirting or real-life dalliances can heighten that sense of je ne sais quoi.

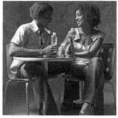

Flirting boosts your self-esteem and is uplifting. Even if it's just harmless fun, it's sure to put a spring in your step.

It's a funny thing, but the best flirters are already in relationships and therefore have a less goal-orientated approach to spreading a few warm smiles. They have nothing to lose, and find it easier to chat with strangers and give out compliments. This is not necessarily a bad thing. Flirting is normal behavior and is even expected in some social situations—for instance, during a bachelorette party. Anthropologists have even suggested that our brains and language abilities have evolved to make us better at attracting sexual partners. Use your charm to give you a boost; it'll improve your sexual confidence.

Flirting is simply about feeling upbeat, smiling, and using body language that conveys positive emotions. In *The Flirt Coach,* Petra Heskell says about flirting, "It is simply about feeling great about who you are and spreading it to other people, which makes them feel great, too." The crucial way to flirt is to use your eyes more. If you're in a social situation, glance around the room and let your eyes linger on

Here's an idea for you... **The next time you're at a social gathering with your partner, pick out the most attractive man in the room and make a point of talking to him animatedly. It's harmless fun, you're aiming to boost your self-confidence, and if you have a lover in tow it'll show him there could be a little competition . . .**

the people you find interesting. Be careful, though, as eye contact is such a powerful way to communicate. Kate Fox says, in her *SIRC Guide to Flirting*, "It is so disturbing that in normal social encounters, we avoid eye contacts of more than one second." Look around the room a few times. If someone returns your interest or, even better, smiles, then you can feel more confident that they're already interested when you do eventually approach them.

If you've looked at a group of men, don't be afraid to approach all of them. Say something like "Anyone got the time?" and if one of them is interested, he'll make it clear. Don't worry about your opening line, as more attention will be focused on your body language (55 percent) than what you actually say (7 percent). If he wants the conversation to continue, he'll show it.

Defining idea... *"There are times not to flirt. When you're sick. When you're with children. When you're on the witness stand."*
JOYCE JILLSON, author

People who like each other have more eye contact than those who don't and tend to stand closer together. When we initiate conversation, it's likely to be in the personal zone (18–48 in), but during a conversation you might draw closer together into the intimate zone (6–18 in). If things get really personal, and you start whispering in each other's ear— the close intimate zone (0–6 in)—it's normally for a special reason. Even if you're avoiding getting too close or keeping your distance, you know

To turn yourself into a red-hot lover, get some tips from IDEA 17, *Giving it some*.

Try another idea...

the conversation's going well when your partner's body language mirrors your own. It's also easier to get closer to someone when you're sitting side by side, as you might at a bar, for instance, than face to face. Look out for body language that is at odds with the facial gestures and words people use, as the body always betrays what's really going through their minds. People often smile to be polite, but if they have their arms or feet crossed the lower part of the body betrays their real emotion, which is insecurity.

In the same way, pay careful attention to your own posture. Don't cross your arms or use body parts to block off your partner; adopting an open, confident, smiling posture makes you seem easier to talk to. Keep your back straight and avoid hunching your shoulders; it makes you seem more outgoing, and makes you look slimmer, too!

Do flirt with people who you stand a chance of getting somewhere with. Striving to get someone's sexual interest and exploring the possibilities of "will we, won't we" is what it's all about. You never know where that spark of passion will lead . . .

"Flirting is a zestful, invigorating pastime. It is the mental equivalent of doing twenty pushups and jogging five miles, since a good flirt must use her brain about three times normal speed."
CYNTHIA HEIMEL, author

Defining idea...

How did it go?

Q   Isn't flirting childish behavior?

A   *It might use the mechanics of playful/childish behavior such as hair flipping, but it's for a serious purpose—sex. Anthropologist Dr. David Givens maintains that being childish is the way people communicate harmlessness. Gray wolves do the same thing, keeping their distance until an encounter becomes sexual; then they behave like puppies. Dr. Givens says, "We still go through the ritual of courtship much like our mammalian ancestors." Just don't howl at the moon or anything!*

Q   Isn't flirting more likely to lead to an affair?

A   *Possibly, but we tend to have affairs with people we know and spend time with, such as colleagues and friends. These are people we'll get to know anyway whatever our approach. There's also a growing trend to have love affairs for greater intimacy rather than sex. Scientists now believe that women are naturally promiscuous like other females across the animal kingdom. Promiscuous women are more likely to get pregnant and if they have an affair, they're twice as likely to be impregnated by their new partner. Around one in seven children have a different biological father than the one they believe is theirs. In England one study looked at women awaiting NHS fertility treatment whose partners were infertile. Amazingly, 25 percent of them became pregnant before they received any treatment . . .*

Porn star protocol

Tried and tested. A fantastic porn star reveals insider secrets on how to have lots of sex—every day, every way.

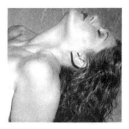

In an exclusive interview, porn star Stormy Daniels gives us the lowdown on her job, her love life, and her top sex tips.

During a phone interview, Stormy proves to be sassy, funny, and quick to answer every question, no matter how personal. She's been working in feature porn films since 2004, exclusively with top porn company Wicked Pictures. She doesn't work in front of the cameras every day, and she also dances, writes, and directs porn films.

A porn shoot is around two to four days of filming and the actors have less sex than you might think. Stormy explains that, with all the waiting and changing positions for different angles, on a typical shoot she'll probably have up to forty minutes of penetrative sex. The sex scenes aren't scripted: "Just the lead-in, like any kind of dialogue that leads up to the kissing. We get to do whatever we want. The director will sit and watch and be like, 'You need to move your leg, we can't see, lean back, look this way, suck in your belly.'" If you're wondering how the actresses seem to be

Here's an idea for you...

Try preparing yourself to be "on call" like a porn star and wait in a carefully appointed dressing room. Get your partner to pop his head in every now and then and bring you drinks . . . you'll be fresh and looking gorgeous, and perhaps waiting for your partner until he says "they" are ready for you will heighten your anticipation.

instantly horny, this is because they get about an hour and a half of foreplay during the lead-in: tell your partner you want to be treated like a porn star and demand the same!

I ask her how she prepares herself for a shoot. "Luckily, I get to pick the people that I work with so I'm almost always looking forward to it," she says. She'll talk to the actors beforehand and agree on what kind of sex they'll get into: "Every time I do a scene with someone I've already worked with, it's easier because you learn with that person, just like in your personal life." Talk to your partner first about positions you're keen to try and come up with a script you can play with. Stormy admits her day job didn't teach her everything; a good relationship helped her to find another sexual dimension: "It wasn't until I was with the person I'm with now that I could have a G-spot orgasm and that's because I was looking in the wrong place!" Every sexual partner can teach you something different, so make more of an effort to reach new sexual highs.

Defining idea...

"But who can we trust to tell us what good sex is? Should we ask people who have a lot of sexual experience, or people who have a lot of research experience?"
KATH ALBURY, author

She doesn't pre-lubricate herself beforehand and says to get herself psyched up she'll go and watch scenes being filmed: "It's kind of like watching real porn!" It especially helps her get in the mood "if there's someone who's really having a good time." The hair and makeup preparation also helps. "It's the same with people in their personal lives; you might not really feel like having sex so much but you go and take a shower and shave your legs and then you're more open to the idea." Stormy suggests that if you feel beautiful before you have sex, you're more likely to enjoy yourself.

Stormy also recommends fantasy and experimentation. "The first time I had sex in front of a mirror was just amazing because I could see something to help me visualize. To this day, this memory is still something I think about when I'm having sex on camera and need to get in the mood." Find your own personal "trigger" fantasy to help you get there.

Her advice to women looking to be a bit more orgasmic is: "Have sex with yourselves to find out what you like. Speak up and say what you want and experiment in bed. If women stop having sex, they stop craving it. But once you get started, the more sex you have, the more you want it."

Enjoy!

If you want to put a few of these ideas into practice, go to IDEA 39, *Girls on film*.

Try another idea...

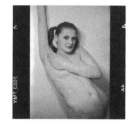

"Maybe there's a little porn star in you. Maybe not. But I can tell you from experience . . . there's a little of you in every porn star."
ANNIE SPRINKLE, sex guru

Defining idea...

How did it go?

Q **Stormy, when you write a porn movie what kinds of things do you put in that maybe a male writer wouldn't?**

A *"Guys mostly want to see people just have sex. Women want to see why these people are having sex. A lot of women need a story line or a setup to get into the mood to follow. It just makes it a little easier for them to digest. When I write I always try to make the sex as hard as possible, but to make the story good enough so that if I took all of the sex scenes out you could still watch the movie and it would make sense." See www.stormyxxx.com or www.wickedpictures.com for details of her movies.*

Q **Any more sex tips?**

A *"The best position for orgasm for most women is woman on top. If your partner's having sex with you, obviously he likes you, otherwise his penis wouldn't be hard, right? So don't be shy. Pornography is a great way to break the ice. You've got to experiment. For the longest time I didn't even like oral sex; for me it was a waste of time. Not to give it, but to get it. I had a partner that just loved doing it and after a while I learned to enjoy it, too." She says, also about her private sex life, "It's about what feels good and not what looks good. But it's hard to get that out of your head, especially if I watch some of my movies and I'm like, 'Aaghh, I will never make that face again!' The only way my job has affected me privately is I have to think at home, 'It doesn't matter, nobody's filming!'"*

26

Be contrary

Put your love life in reverse gear. If you avoid sex, chase it. If there's a position you love, don't do it. Courting frustration could be just the thing you need to drive you over the edge.

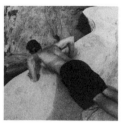

Being intimate is a double-edged sword. Sometimes it brings you too close and you need to be a bit more sexually ruthless to enjoy getting off.

Over time it's almost inevitable for a couple's sex life to decrease in frequency. Often we're simply unrealistic about our sexual expectations because our culture is saturated with images of sex and romantic longing. We feel like we should want more, and this unfocused yearning can lead to people seeking out affairs. It's possible to be in an endless cycle of falling in love, getting disillusioned, meeting someone else, and repeating the whole cycle; Elizabeth Taylor once described herself as "addicted to love."

In reality the thing we have to deal with most when we grapple with sexual problems is our own psyche. During sex we have to open ourselves up to our vulnerabilities. Psychotherapist Dr. Michael Bader says in *Arousal: The Secret Logic of*

Here's an idea for you...

Ask your partner to describe your contribution to your lovemaking; make a careful note of what he says, then for a limited time reverse this behavior. If he normally initiates sex, you do it for a change. You'll have sex sessions using completely different methods and techniques than the ones you're used to, and perhaps you'll be pleasantly surprised!

Sexual Fantasies, "We go to bed naked in more ways than one." We all carry insecurities with us that have been with us from childhood, and at first a new sexual liaison gives us a chance to work against this. If a woman has grown up feeling physically inferior to her beautiful mother, she might initially take refuge in a relationship with an especially attractive man. However, over time, her old insecurities will emerge and return to plague her, and this is why so many couples start to experience sexual problems after the "honeymoon period" that were not at first apparent.

Some couples say they have less sex but it's more intimate; however, this has its own problems. The more intimate you become, the more you're aware of your partner's frailties. Dr. Bader also says, "As couples get to know each other, their deeper awareness of each other's vulnerabilities can become their undoing. The other's inhibitions and the shame upon which they rest begin to wear down spontaneity and passion. We are just too close, too identified with our inhibited partner, to escape the experience." It's important for you to have a certain degree of sexual ruthlessness and sometimes we all need some kind of emotional distance (via fantasy or physical space) in order to be able to switch off and concentrate on our own sexual needs.

If your sex life is nothing to write home about, try deliberately avoiding it for a while. If something's on tap you take it for granted. See how long you can go without having sex

Play around with who sexually dominates the other—check out IDEA 9, *Point of entry.*

Try another idea...

together. It's a good idea not to stop all physical activity: you could try masturbating separately and telling each other all about it when you do get together. The idea is to get you hot, but you can still agree whether to postpone sex or not—and maybe tomorrow when you eventually succumb to passion it'll be even better. Sometimes being frustrated, that feeling of suppressed longing, leads to the best sex of all, so it's worth waiting until you just can't hold back.

To objectify your partner a little, you could also try playing around with sexual fantasy. Get him to dress up a little differently or speak to you in bed in a different voice. You're trying to think of him erotically as a means to give you great sex, rather than your soul mate with lots of problems he wants to talk over.

Over time we can desexualize our partners, so now's the time to inject some throbbing desire into the proceedings. It could be that he's treating you gently when you really want to be ravaged, so try talking dirty and see if this makes it easier for you to get excited. Force yourself to expose your throbbing desires. That's it—get down and dirty and sex up your relationship.

"An absence, the decline of a dinner invitation, an unintentional coldness, can accomplish more than all the cosmetics and beautiful dresses in the world."
MARCEL PROUST

Defining idea...

How did it go?

Q   I find the idea of being "sexually ruthless" ridiculous. My partner would never take me seriously. Now what?

A   *Aha! That's the problem—you're just too close. You could try putting a physical distance between you for a while, go on vacation with a girlfriend, or visit your parents/friends and see if this helps. Some couples find moving to a long-distance relationship makes for more quality time, even though they see each other less. You need to find some way to relate to your partner as a sex object again. Choosing not to have sex for an agreed time is a pretty easy option and it's cheaper than therapy!*

Q   Isn't the whole point of sex to become intimate?

A   *Yes, up to a point. As Dr. Bader says, "The paradox of sexual arousal is that in order for us to experience it intensely, we have to be able to both connect with our partner and to take him or her for granted." This is a problem common in the lesbian community where couples are so sensitive to each other that it desexualizes their relationship, a phenomenon known as "lesbian death bed." When sociologists Philip Blumstein and Pepper Schwartz did the American Couples' Survey, which looked at heterosexual, married, unmarried, gay, and lesbian couples, those in lesbian relationships had the least sex of all: 47 percent had sex once a month or less.*

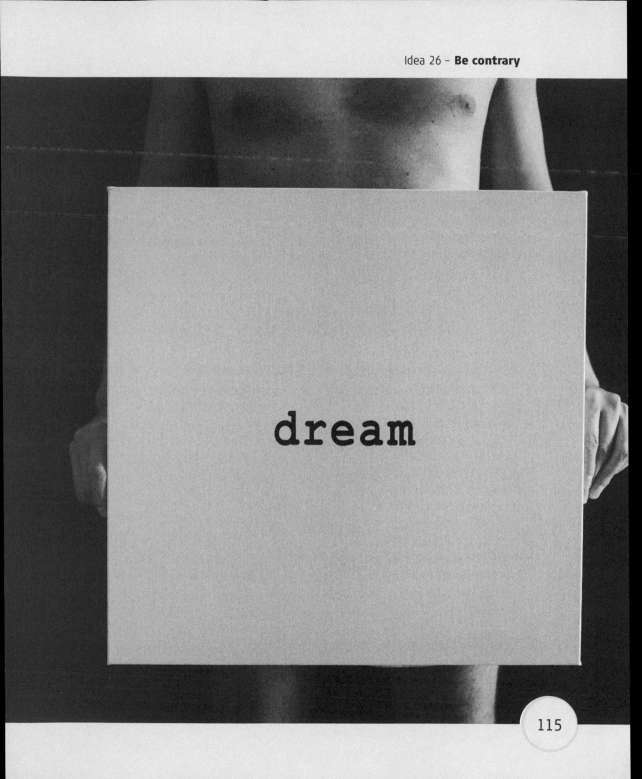

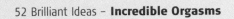

27

Indecent proposal

Do you indulge in secret fantasies? How to put a finger on that fancy.

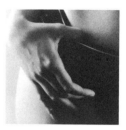

Fantasizing is normal human behavior. Once you've worked out what makes you tick, you've got a fast-track route to orgasms.

All of us fantasize—it could be about winning the lottery or dating Orlando Bloom—and sexual fantasies that arouse us are no different. In 1968 when Nancy Friday was researching her first book on women's fantasies, *My Secret Garden,* no psychologist was willing to accept that "normal" women had sexual fantasies, but now researchers say there is no gender difference between male and female fantasizing. Harold Leitenberg and Kris Henning in *Sexual Fantasy*, their mammoth project, show that women's fantasies help them to overcome taboos and real-life problems. They turn off our inner censor and act as a coping strategy to get rid of guilt and negative emotions. Just in case you think there's something pervy about doing it, actually the reverse is true, as Leitenberg says, "The people who have the most sexual problems fantasize least." Those who indulge in erotic fantasy have sex more frequently, have a wider sexual repertoire, and have more sexual partners. There's really no excuse not to do it!

Here's an idea for you...

To delve deeper into his sexual psyche, get your partner to write his secret fantasies on your back with a lip liner pencil. You won't be able to see them unless you look in a mirror (and then you have to be able to read backward) so his secret is safe unless he can trust you enough to reveal all. If you only get part of the way in one session, take a bath and get him to wash it all off.

Women think about sex at least four and a half times a day. The trick is to hold on to some of these fleeting images so you can make use of them. Keep a dream/mood diary, and write down things and people that arouse a flicker of sexual interest. The trick is to find out what turns you on. There could be a theme or specific activity that gets you going. (And it could be anything: one Nerve.com writer gets turned on by the twirls Wonder Woman does as she transforms.) Try browsing websites like www.cliterati.co.uk or www.literotic.com. They're free and you can search by topic. Don't be alarmed if you find yourself turned on by things you'd never want to do in real life (like incest or gangbang fantasies). Often we're drawn to these as coping mechanisms and they represent a desire to attract attention—in fantasy life it's common to sexualize these basic desires. Fantasizing about it doesn't mean you want to enact it, that's why they're called fantasies. It's not important why something turns you on, only finding out what works for you.

Defining idea...

"I've always suspected that women had richer, wilder fantasies than men."
HENRY MILLER

Some women find their wildest thoughts are actually quite mundane. Don't worry if your fantasy isn't exotic, as the most common one is sex with a current or past lover. In addition, Leitenberg and Henning say the three most common "flavors" of fantasy are using novel/forbidden imagery, scenes of sexual irresistibility, and dominance/submissive fantasies. When we are "done to" and dominated it relieves us of any sexual responsibility; we don't have to feel guilty about anything.

Once you've mastered being able to turn yourself on using fantasy, add another technique to your love-making repertoire— see IDEA 6, *Shivering with anticipation.*

Try another idea...

To get more acquainted with your secret fantasies, browse books, websites, and erotic films for inspiration. Try to spend some time in the week on your own, safe behind a locked door. Some find sanctuary in the bathroom, where they can sip a glass of wine as they soak in the bath and let their mind wander. Let your thoughts take you wherever they want to go, and resist the urge to self-censor.

The next step is masturbation. Ideally you've titillated yourself with erotic thoughts first, as once your body has responded it's easier to play with yourself when you are moist. The joint action of fantasizing and masturbation is a double turn-on. Many women use the same fantasies they use to masturbate during sex with their partner, too. Some lovers divulge all their sexual secrets, but it's up to you to decide whether or not to tell your partner everything: you can always tell them a minor predilection and reserve your hottest, wettest fantasies for your mind only!

"There is a boundary to men's passions when they act from feelings; but none when they are under the influence of imagination."
JOHN BARRYMORE

Defining idea...

How did it go?

Q **I never have sexual fantasies. Is there something wrong with me?**

A *Well, about 5 percent of men and women say they never have erotic fantasies. Some researchers think they just don't admit to having them, or don't acknowledge the sexual side of things when they do emerge. We can't really be certain what we dream about, can we? Psychiatrist Ethel Person, author of* By Force of Fantasy, *reckons those who claim not to fantasize just get their kicks elsewhere. Don't worry about not fantasizing, but it wouldn't hurt to try letting your mind wander on the wild side a bit more.*

Q **If I let loose with my fantasies, isn't there a danger that I could act them out in real life?**

A *No. Engaging with the fantasy in your head seems to take the power out of it. Although rape fantasies (as a victim) are common, the act is rare in real life. Only 22 percent of child molesters actually claim to have engaged in sexual fantasies about children before their first molestation. About one in four of us feel guilty about our fantasies: in studies 51 percent of women fantasized about being forced to have sex, and some feminists feel uncomfortable about it. The thing to do is accept your fantasies as just that: fantasies.*

28

A hairy situation

The nitty-gritty essentials of personal hygiene: how to remove hair, plus ingenious tips for beautifying the pudenda zone.

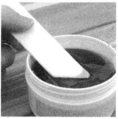

The jury's out on whether it's better for your bush to be au naturel or not. Whatever you do, do it to increase your sexual confidence and to boost your body image.

Some people prefer pubic hair, others do not. The writer Mil Millington has argued fiercely that we should ban the "Brazilian" wax: "Aesthetically, very few things are less appealing than the plucked-chicken-flesh look of barren genitals." Also, Violet Blue, the sex educator, argues in favor of shaving: "For many of us the result was an unforgettable feeling of silky-smooth skin, sensitive to the touch, with all of the bare skin's nerve endings at full attention." The way we present ourselves celebrates our diversity. Removing hair, or coloring it, is an easy way to do this.

If you don't want to actually remove any hair, use a pair of nail scissors for an overall trim. If you want to depilate for a V shape, you could consider the common methods: a bikini line wax, shaving, or a depilation cream. It's best to have waxing done at a salon, but you will need at least six weeks' growth. It is

Here's an idea for you...

Remove a little bit of your pubic hair near your stomach and beautify yourself. You could use a stick-on tattoo or diamante, or draw something with an eye pencil. Spruce yourself up and you'll feel more sexually confident.

painful (avoid doing it when you are premenstrual and feel pain more intensely) but it will be smooth for around four weeks. Avoid taking a bath or shower after waxing, and exfoliate with a loofah or body scrub every few days to prevent a rash as the hairs start to come back.

People with slow hair growth could consider depilatory creams, especially for the bikini area. These are also good when waxing is growing out and you are in between stages. You'll need to leave the cream on for around ten minutes and won't be able to use soap in the area right away (not recommended just before he goes down on you). Shaving is quickest, but all methods can result in prickly regrowth.

To remove more of the hair, or the whole lot, you could try a Brazilian wax or shaving. It's best to have a Brazilian done at a speciality salon; it will take around half an hour and all the parts of your vulva, including your anus, will be waxed. Afterward you can have the area decorated with Swarovski crystals—tiny gems with adhesive backs. Alternatively, use temporary tattoos.

You can also shave yourself at home. It's best to soften the hair first by taking a bath or lying a wet cloth over it. Use conditioner on your pubic hair to pre-soften. Cut the hair short with scissors or with an electric beard trimmer. (First timers might want to try an overall trim first to see how it feels—I promise this will not prickle the skin.) It's important to sit or lie near a mirror so you can see what you are doing. Use shaving cream and shave in the direction the hair grows.

If you enjoy any cosmetic changes you've made to your pudenda region, why not immortalize them? See IDEA 39, *Girls on film*.

Try another idea...

Have a little bowl of water ready to dip the razor into after every stroke. Use a towel to wipe away excess foam so you can see what you are doing. On tricky areas use hold the skin taut, or even ask your partner to help you and make it an erotic experience. Taking all the hair off takes practice. Violet Blue says that shaving your anus is difficult because you can't see it. She suggests "turning around and bending over completely, so you're looking through your legs at your butt in the mirror, and use your free hand to pull your buttocks aside." Use a soothing cream or zinc oxide lotion afterward.

Other methods include laser surgery, which needs repeated sessions; sugaring; and threading. Ask your beautician about these. Some people show off their handiwork with a tattoo or genital piercing. You can also dye the pubic hair with henna and cut it into shapes. If it feels good, flaunt it.

"Body hair is, after all, Mother Nature's own bossy-boots burka, covering up the bits she deems too attractive to be on show, and it never hurts to show who's boss."
JULIE BURCHILL

Defining idea...

How did it go?

Q **After I shaved my pubic hair off for the first time, I hated the look of my vulva. I'd never noticed before how big my vaginal lips are. Is this just me?**

A *No, they vary considerably. Too many of us worry about not being the norm (porn models are routinely altered with cosmetic surgery or Photoshopped to look uniform). Take a mirror and spend some time looking at yourself. If this is the first time you have done this, get used to it; us women have to go out of our way to get a look down there. Betty Dodson has a gallery of genitalia on her website, www.bettydodson.com, so check that out. People are invited to send in their own pictures—go on, I dare you!*

Q **I like being completely smooth, but not the painful regrowth. Is there anything I can do to prevent this?**

A *When you get rid of hair on other parts of your body (legs, for instance) do you also get a rash? If so, then you probably have sensitive skin. Some people are more prone than others to itching and sensitivity, although die-hards say that over time it gets easier (they would). You can be allergic to the soap/shaving foam or moisturizer product you are using; try hypoallergenic versions. Experiment with the different methods. Afterward, don't wear tight clothes for a few days and use cortisone cream to reduce swelling, but don't overuse as it can thin the skin.*

29
Ouch!

Is it me, or did that feel wrong? A little troubleshooting for those oh-so-sensitive areas.

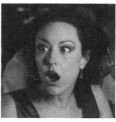

The best lover in the world can't light your fire if there's something amiss down south. It may not even be an infection; plain old vulval sensitivity is more common than you think.

Because our vaginas are inside our bodies it's harder for us to examine ourselves if things feel a bit off. Add the guilt and shame that many feel at the prospect of a ripening sexual infection and you've got a recipe for disaster. A survey in the *Journal of the American Medical Association* in 1999 suggested that 14 percent experienced problems with sexual arousal (lack of vaginal lubrication) and 7 percent had pain during intercourse. Oh, and add to that the 22 percent who complained of low sexual desire (and, of course, painful sex today is likely to lead to sexual dysfunction tomorrow) and you can see that feeling plain old uncomfortable takes the joy out of sex. Although yeast infections (candida albicans) often causes soreness, along with STDs, the most common reason for pain during sex is actually vulval vestibulitis, which translates as soreness down south. Unfortunately, doctors don't really understand its causes—it's most frequently caused by yeast infection or allergic dermatitis, but this part of the body is just as likely to be susceptible to dryness and itching.

Here's an idea for you...

If you have recurrent sensitivity in the vaginal or anal area, try using a sitz bath. Run a shallow bath, sit for fifteen minutes, and rinse off. It should bring down any swelling and is good for soothing delicate skin.

It goes without saying that you should visit an OB/GYN (obstetrician/gynecologist) for a checkup about as often as you go to the dentist. If you feel any soreness, go for a checkup. At the clinic they will open your vagina with a speculum and take swabs, which are tested the same day; they will also grow bacteria from the swabs in a laboratory for further analysis. Often women with a yeast infection get a false negative at first, but a week later it can show up in the lab. Don't assume that you'll be able to "tell" if you have an infection: herpes can manifest itself as strips of red, sore skin rather than ulcers, and most women don't know if they have chlamydia, which currently constitutes 40 percent of the caseload at OB/GYN clinics.

If microbiological testing shows the presence of a yeast infection, you can take oral medication, pessaries, and creams. For extra soreness use hydrocortisone cream, which also relieves itching and inflammation. You will be given treatment for any sexual infection. The problem comes if you get the all clear but it still hurts.

Defining idea...

"Pain is such an uncomfortable feeling that even a tiny amount of it is enough to ruin every enjoyment."
WILL ROGERS

If tests are negative for yeast or any other STD, it could be that you are allergic to a bath or laundry product. Avoid perfumed soaps and use hypoallergenic brands or simple aqueous cream. Don't use bath additives—add a cup of salts instead. One thing most people don't realize is that you could be allergic to the shampoo or conditioner you use to wash your hair; for this reason, avoid washing your hair in the bath. The golden rule is anything that might be remotely perfumed should be kept away from delicate areas, and that includes talcum powder, vaginal douches, and deodorant sprays, and perfumed sanitary pads. Culprits for sensitivity come from all sorts of places; it is even possible to be allergic to the dyes in colored toilet paper. Some women are also allergic to their partner's semen.

Encourage acid conditions in the vagina by using a mildly acidic gel or using a probiotic supplement; you can also eat/apply natural live yogurt. In her *Ultimate Guide to Cunnilingus* Violet Blue says, "The natural healthy vagina should have a slightly pungent, sweet odor, similar to that of plain yogurt: that's because the same bacteria, lactobacilli, exist in both environments." Avoid too much sugar and alcohol, which can trigger a bacteria overgrowth. Are you allergic to rubber? If so, use Avanti condoms and non-latex sex toys.

Finally, if in doubt, keep it out: never have sex if you are not lubricated. Always monitor any vaginal/anal soreness. Prevention is better than cure, so give the gateway to your pleasure a little TLC.

For more tips on understanding your sexual health, see IDEA 3, *Sticky fingers.*

Try another idea...

"It is easier to find men who will volunteer to die, than to find those who are willing to endure pain with patience."
JULIUS CAESAR

Defining idea...

127

How did it go?

Q   Even though my boyfriend gives me a lot of hot foreplay, sometimes I find sex is still painful. What should I do?

A   *Men know when they're aroused because they get an erection; it's much harder for women to know if they're really ready for sex. Research at Amsterdam University into female arousal has shown that it's highly complex; although a vagina should become moist from fluids on the genital walls and get longer and expand, many of the test subjects in the experiment responded unpredictably. Dr. Ellen Laan said, "They were unaware if they're lubricating properly or not." It's hard for you to assess if you are really ready, so play safe and use extra lubricant first. You can also put a blob of it on the end of your boyfriend's penis for ease of entry. If you still have problems, visit an OB/GYN and give yourself a little vacation from vaginal sex—there are other possibilities to keep you both happy!*

Q   If there's no medical reason for pain during sex, does that mean it can't be treated?

A   *No. In a recent article, "Dyspareunia and Vulvar Disease," researchers Marin, et al., found that in the beginning there was an original cause for the painful sex, which led to a subsequent low level of lubrication that made the problem worse. However, whatever their original problem, all the women needed the same treatment—avoid having sex if it hurts.*

30

Dosing up

The latest on massage oils, potions, and pills. The appliance of science plus the return of an old favorite, energy-enhancing vitamins.

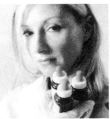

We've always had things to pep up a flagging libido. These days, as well as pills and potions, there are mechanical devices and medical techniques to do the job...

Throughout history, aphrodisiacs have been popular as a food, drink, drug, scent, or mechanical device. Named after the Greek goddess of love, Aphrodite, most of them simply resemble the sexual organs they are meant to stimulate. A common one is ginseng, and—guess what—its male flowers resemble a penis and its female ones a vagina. Other popular ones include anchovies, rhinoceros horn, celery, and oysters—I'll leave you to work these ones out! The good old *Kama Sutra*, as well as containing how-to positions, also details sensuous recipes, for example: "An ointment made of the fruit of the asteracantah longifolia will contract the yoni of a Hastini or Elephant woman, and this contraction lasts for one night." Even today there are a plethora of "natural products" that claim to build up libido, despite the fact that the FDA way back in 1989 pooh-poohed manufacturers' claims that any of the over-the-counter potions work.

Here's an idea for you...

Try Femi-X, the new exciting product from Medic House. The multipack contains herbal pills designed to naturally increase female libido, and it comes complete with an educational CD and a cool DVD featuring clitoris-friendly positions. It's available at pharmacies or from www.femi-x.com.

Of course, since 1998 we've had Viagra. It can work wonders for men, but it doesn't do so much for women. Viagra is not a sexual stimulant; it works by helping to increase the blood flow—a godsend in certain sensitive areas, but it's probably effective for only one in ten women.

For the more practical, there are also rubbing lotions like L-arginine amino-acid cream, which helps athletes to build muscles—and is reputed to give better arousal and orgasm. Some women swear by testosterone therapy; in a trial reported in the *New England Journal of Medicine*, women given extra testosterone found their arousal rate increased by two to three times. Research is ongoing for testosterone patches like Intrinsa that increase localized blood flow to the genital area and are likely to come on the market soon; they're especially suitable for women going through menopause. A new trend in cosmetic surgery is plumping up the G-spot with injections. Devotees say it increases sensations, but it has to be done every few months, so I hope it's worth the effort!

Defining idea...

"The mind is the most potent aphrodisiac there is."
JOHN RENNER, consumer researcher

Surgeon Stuart Meloy has developed an electronic spinal implant that makes use of neurally augmented surgery to implant an electrode into the spinal area that attaches to a device, the orgasmatron, which stimulates orgasm. In tests, women who had never had an orgasm were able to experience one. The treatment costs $17,000 and Dr. Meloy is the only person in the world offering this service. A temporary one-week implant costs $3,800 and makes for a romantic vacation; for more details see www.aipmnc.com. If you like science fiction, computer scientist Kevin Warwick and his wife seem to be having the kind of cybersex we see in the movies. They both have surgically inserted computer chips so that they can stream their consciousness together for that mental and physical connection; check out their website at www.kevinwarwick.com.

Psychologists reckon that when it comes to the body, it really is a question of mind over matter: see IDEA 20, *Mind games*.

Try another idea...

Don't forget that what's good for your general health does wonders for your libido, too. If you don't feel the urge, check your basic vitamin intake. Are you eating the recommended five portions of fruit and veggies a day? Taking a basic multivitamin is a good thing to do (although pregnant women or those planning to conceive should take special prenatal vitamins—too much vitamin A can harm a fetus). If this doesn't work, Dr. Sarah Brewer suggests taking evening primrose oil, as it contains essential fatty acids that balance out the sex hormones. Saint-John's-Wort may also help if tiredness is turning you off. There are also "prosexual" health supplements to experiment with, including ginkgo (boosts circulation), damiana (increases nerve sensitivity), and muira puama ("potency wood"). From folklore and natural remedies to Frankenstein-like devices, we are pretty much spoiled for choice!

"The idea that you can just give someone a pill and they'll be interested in sex is like putting a Band-Aid on a tumor."
DR. JANICE EPP, clinical psychologist

Defining idea...

How did it go?

Q   You didn't mention many of the products I've seen advertised that promise to enhance desire. Aren't they worth a look, too?

A   *There are lots out there, but that doesn't mean they're any good. John Renner from the Consumer Health Information Research Institute says companies promote their products using a "blatant snake-oil approach" and that a fraudulent love potion industry exists where products can be unsafe to use, as well as being ineffective.*

Q   My partner wants to have sex more often than I do. Do I really need to use some of these products/techniques or is there something wrong with me?

A   *There's probably nothing wrong with you if your general health is OK (you're not generally feeling tired, having lots of headaches, and so on). No one has really worked out what level of activity is "normal." Every individual's sex drive is as individual as her taste in food or level of sport activity. Clinical psychologist and sex therapist Sandra Pertot says, "The pressure in therapy is most commonly on the person with the lower sex drive to pick up the pace." The media has stereotyped the image of highly sexed women, which puts a lot of pressure and guilt on women to think that they should be feeling more highly sexed than they need to be. By all means, make use of these tips if they work for you, but don't be pressured into assuming you should be feeling horny twenty-four hours a day.*

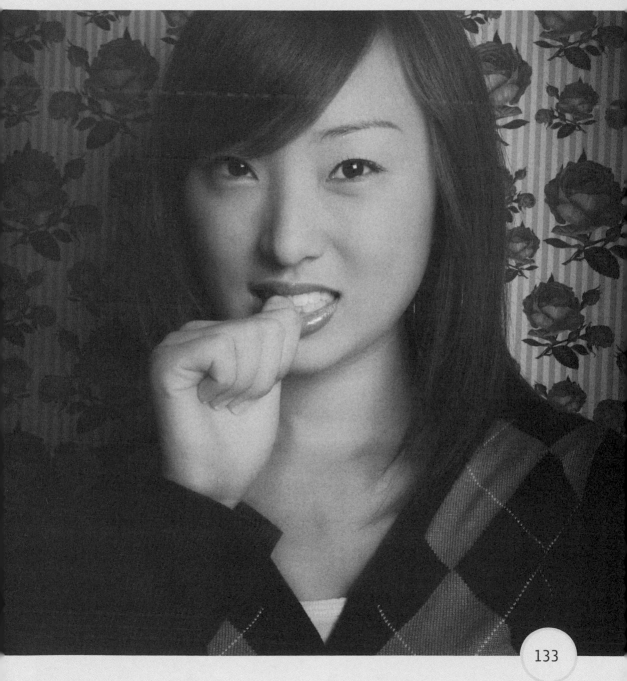

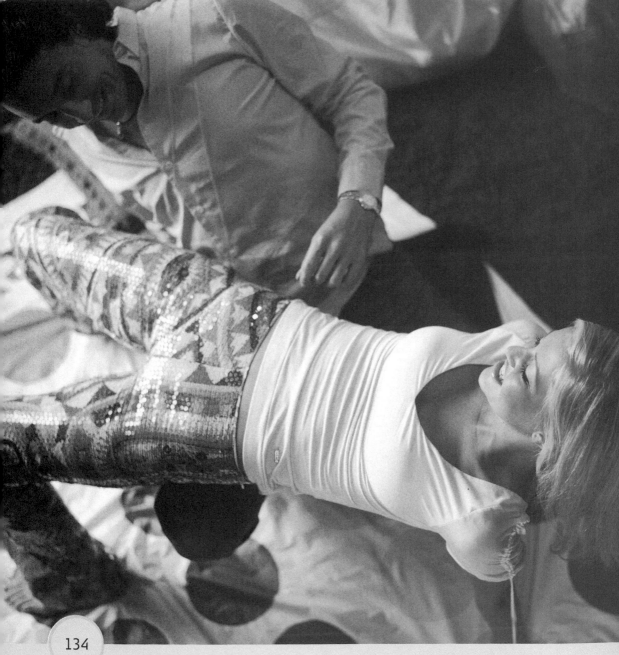

31

Coming back after turning off

Perhaps you've had a baby or other life-changing experience. If you just never feel in the mood anymore, reconnecting with your sexual self is the first stage.

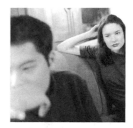

Our permanent sexual availability is almost unique in the animal kingdom, but that doesn't mean we always have to be rampant or indulge in it daily.

Believe it or not, the clitoris doesn't have a real function and female orgasm isn't really necessary for conception. Some women (around 10 percent) claim never to orgasm, and around 40 percent experience some sexual dysfunction, yet if we're lacking on the old libido front we immediately assume there's a problem. Perhaps we don't feel sexy because we simply don't need it.

Orgasms during sexual contact are not always necessary. If a woman is aroused and experiences intimacy with her partner, that is often good enough. Unfortunately, in a world where sex sells, not having enough sex makes us feel guilty or inadequate.

In certain situations it's normal to avoid sex. If you've not been enjoying the sex you've been having, or if it's become painful or emotionally strained, it's only

Here's an idea for you... **Take a warm bath, pop in a bath bomb, lie back, and put on a face pack, and drink lots of fresh juices as you chill out in scented water. You'll be less stressed (a libido buster) and the warm water improves blood circulation and gets things moving more quickly. Try masturbating with your shower spray or a waterproof dildo on your clit; a very clean way to get horny.**

natural that you're not going to be lining up to repeat the experience. After a miscarriage or abortion, you'll also have to deal with the hormonal downturn before you even grapple with the emotional scars. After having a baby, you'll be physically more tired, have the pain of an episiotomy scar, and breastfeeding can make you as dry as a bone—it lowers your levels of estrogen (less of that lovely lubricant). It's not surprising that sex is problematic at these times. Professor Lesley Regan says in *Your Pregnancy Week By Week*, "It is estimated that more than 50 percent of couples have not returned to their pre-pregnancy sexual activity one year after the birth of their first child."

The good news is that it's exactly when you're in this take it or leave it cul-de-sac that you have the restraint necessary to pick up some new moves and techniques. When you're under the thrall of passion, you're responding instinctively; having sex with your brain in control might not be so bad after all.

Defining idea... *"The desire for intercourse is the genius of the genus."*
ARTHUR SCHOPENHAUER

Go back to "third base" and initiate sessions devoted exclusively to foreplay. Leave your clothes on and fool around. Talk and snuggle up with your partner whenever you can. Grab the opportunity to find out if something about your sexual tastes has changed.

If the vaginal area is sore or out-of-bounds, try responding to breast, anal, or foot fondling instead. Touching, kissing, hugging, and stroking are all just as good as sex (ask a foot fetishist!). Don't forget it's easier to bite the bullet and give your partner oral sex or cuddle him while he whacks off to a porn video than feel guilty. Ignoring sex won't make it go away.

For the latest libido pick-me-ups and a little scientific help to recapture your desire, turn to IDEA 30, *Dosing Up*.

Try another idea...

Of course, what you want to hear is how to flip the magic button—you don't want comfort when there's that ideal of multiple orgasms for ever after. But if we're tired or stressed, the first thing that shrinks is our libido. In addition, how you feel at the outset of a make-out session is no indication of how you'll feel after lots of foreplay (I can't count the times I've said "Not tonight, I'm not in the mood" only to scream rampantly later).

Trust yourself and give yourself time to enjoy anything that comes your way. And while you're at it, give yourself some extra sleep to make sure that simple tiredness is not destroying your mood. Don't forget that most of the time we're in bed just to sleep, so it's natural to associate this space more with the land of nod than exhilarating thrills. Experiment with the sofa, or maybe a rug on the floor in front of the fire. Hey, if you want to go crazy, get some "sex" furniture that makes it easier to try out the positions of the *Kama Sutra*.

Defining idea...

"A knowing woman's work is never done
To get a lover if she hasn't one,
But as I had them eating from my hand
And as they'd yielded me their gold and land,
Why then take trouble to provide them pleasure
Unless to profit and amuse my leisure?"
GEOFFREY CHAUCER'S *Wife of Bath*

How did it go?

Q   My husband and I have been together for twenty years and there's just no spark. We're best friends, not lovers. Even the idea of foreplay seems silly! What now?

A   *Being best friends with your husband sounds great! There is some evidence to suggest that after a certain amount of time couples no longer feel attracted to each other. As far back as 1891 the sociologist Edward Westermarck, in* The History of Human Marriage, *suggested this is why we avoid incest by choice: we're simply not attracted to people we spend lots of time with. In 1995 Arthur Wolf published a paper reexamining Westermarck's theory, which he applied to 14,000 Chinese women. Those who had been raised within the family to marry their "brothers" from infancy were nearly three times as likely to divorce as those who met on their wedding day! Break this cycle; try to get a bit of distance. Spend weekends apart, initiate dirty telephone calls. Make your time together precious, rather than taking each other for granted.*

Q   I'm a woman in my forties. Isn't it normal for desire to drop off as you get older?

A   *No, quite the opposite. Although Hollywood would have you believe that only the young feel sexy, in reality sex is more important to older couples. Reader's Digest published a poll undertaken by ICM in 2003 showing couples in the 24–34 age group were least concerned with sex. Men and women in the 35–44 age group had more interest in good sex.*

32

Your sexual profile

You never forget your first time, right? Do you have a "template" that traces your sexual predilections? Do you have your panties in a twist about something?

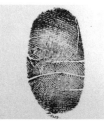

Figuring out how you've been sexually imprinted gives you a chance to buck the trend and avoid bad sex and abusive relationships.

Our first sexual partners are usually the most formative, as through them we create a sexual template that largely defines what we see as desirable. For many women the man who they lose their virginity to is important, but the template could also be based on a romantic attachment that never went beyond a kiss. Everyone has a mental idea of what they think of as sexy, but it's a little disconcerting to deconstruct this and work out that because of a foray with a floppy-headed fool in 1988 you're still pursuing Byronic types with dark hair. This explains why all Rod Stewart's significant others look the same: the gentleman obviously prefers leggy blondes.

Given that first-time sex can be a bit hit and miss, it's a little scary to think that this can affect our whole perception of sex for years to come. What we think of as our personal sexual predilections are probably inherited from a formative sexual blueprint. Sex columnist Tracey Cox says in "Why Your First Lover Affects You for

Here's an idea for you...

Try to work out your sexual template. Go through old photos of your lovers. What characteristics do you find attractive? Now think about what negative traits these lovers brought with them. If you could go back in time, what things would you change? Mentally revise your checklist. It could be that over time you go for the security of someone in gainful employment rather than a wannabe rock star.

Life": "We usually pick our first partners carefully (if not sensibly) but few, if any of us, realize how strongly we'll be influenced by his physical characteristics and love-making style."

This makes a good argument for choosing a good man for the job, but for many of us it's too late; we have to live with our blueprints. If your first sexual experience was negative, it's probably going to be harder for you to pick someone more compatible because you're working off a script based on the original loser.

The trick is to work out what's going on by looking at your past conquests and making a mental checklist of similarities. You'll probably find that if your friends know your exes they'll be better at spotting characteristics, so it's worth asking their advice. The aim is to widen your potential dating quota by challenging the stereotype of what you think is "sexy." We make assumptions about other potential partners based on our blueprint all the time (as they do with us) and it makes life easier if we can extend our repertoire a little wider than Rod Stewart does, and feel attracted to dating people with a wider cultural and physical makeup.

Defining idea...

"First love is a kind of vaccination which saves a man from catching the complaint a second time."
HONORÉ DE BALZAC

Similarly with your sexual preferences, if you look harder at what was imprinted into you those first couple of times, you'll find you've been unconsciously replicating this. Did he turn you on to rough sex? What's your preferred way to kiss? This is especially important because if you've had a bad experience you may have been avoiding things that could give you pleasure with the right partner. Some women's experiences were abusive, so not having decent orgasms is the least of their problems, but the principle is the same. Work against the grain.

If you're a bad-boy magnet, check out IDEA 44, *The rake*, for why you find this type alluring.

Try another idea...

Now you have to separate the things that turn you on independently from your formative blueprint. Perhaps at the age of twenty-five you suddenly decided you liked having your toes sucked during foreplay or you couldn't get enough of erotic massage. Probe into your fantasy life. Even though external stimuli, like porn and fashion photography, attempt to shape our preferences, there's some core sense of your sexual identity that is unique to you. Getting in touch with this will help get rid of the clutter of secondhand imprinting and clear the way for the fastest route to orgasms. Think of it as emotional spring cleaning. Keep a dream diary and encourage yourself to get into those wandering sexual fantasies. You're floating in a rich inner fantasy life; don't you want to know what truly turns you on?

"I know nothing about sex because I was always married."
ZSA ZSA GABOR

Defining idea...

141

How did
it go?

Q **If women have had a bad experience, why do they go for the same type of guy again?**

A *Usually we find a way to normalize a bad experience, especially if it happens over a long period of time. It's astonishing how kidnap victims can identify positively with their oppressors in a matter of days. National surveys estimate that up to 30 percent of women treated in emergency rooms are victims of domestic violence. In 2005 Susan Darker-Smith suggested that fairy tales like Cinderella can make little girls more likely to stay in abusive relationships later on because they identify with the submissive heroines. Around one in three of us will encounter physical abuse in a relationship, and the surveys haven't even touched on negative sexual imprinting yet!*

Q **If I'm into weird stuff, is that my ex's fault?**

A *Yes and no. Sometimes we like something only temporarily. However, some people have unfortunate sexual predilections, which means they can only get turned on in situations that are probably not going to happen with a reciprocal partner they're not paying. Some of them would probably change this if they could, but they can't. Somehow it's wired in.*

33

Let yourself go

Challenge yourself to lose one of your inhibitions. Actors train by caressing each other blindfolded in their underwear. Perhaps you need to do something adventurous to really reach that plateau.

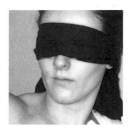

Our fears and pleasures are close allies. Learning how to push yourself in one of these directions helps you to become more of a "sensation seeker."

Some women find their orgasm experience is elusive or thwarted because part of them is holding back. In fact, the definition of anorgasmia (the inability to have an orgasm) is the involuntary inhibition of the orgasmic reflex. It's mostly the fear of being out of control that can prevent or muffle a perfectly good orgasm. Think of it as a phobia, a bit like a fear of spiders; we aren't born with this as an innate fear, but we can be conditioned into learning it.

Like anyone with inhibitions, the most positive way to put such doubts behind you is to concentrate on other things. It's a mistake to think people who are shy are suffering from low self-esteem; they behave that way because they're overly

Here's an idea for you... **This weekend you're going to try something daring. What about caving, riding a roller coaster, go-carting, or learning to dive? Book yourself a session or a class and just go for it. If you find the experience nerve-racking at first, just imagine your sense of achievement (and relief) when you've completed it. Now think about doing the same in bed.**

concerned with their self-image. If you're feeling nervous about not being able to come you can counter this by focusing on your partner's pleasure, the music that's playing, the beautiful sunset, whatever. By switching the attention away from you, it'll make it easier to relax and let your hair down. Because of the longer time it takes for women to get aroused, there's sometimes too much emphasis on our needs. On the one hand, it's great to get the attention, but if your partner makes your pleasure the center of the sex experience, it can also make you feel more self-conscious and less likely to lose your inhibitions.

Think like Marilyn Monroe. Although she rarely climaxed, she was enthusiastic about sex and cared deeply about her partner's needs. Stop thinking of yourself as a spectator and just go with the flow; at a nightclub if you thought consciously of all the moves you were making while dancing, you'd stop yourself from moving. Let your body fall into its own rhythm or, if you feel too embarrassed to buck your lower body, choose static positions like the doggy style where you can relax and enjoy being "done to."

Defining idea... *"Adventures come to the adventurous."*
ENID BLYTON

It can also help to focus on one sensation, like the feel of your hair whipping back, the movement of your skin, your partner's face. Concentrate on any fleeting physical aspect to take your mind off things. Don't be afraid to moan and do at least try to look like you're having a ball. If you think positive, you're much more likely to get the result you want. Top athletes train by visualizing goals as if they were already achieved and, strangely, these mental tricks seem to work. Yep, it is possible to kid yourself into having a real orgasm; sex therapist Barbara Keesling says that if you mimic the throes of orgasm you're more likely to really climax.

Work on smoothing out some of your inhibitions. These don't have to be sexual; if you only step out of the house with full makeup on, trying doing without any. If there's something you dread doing, try it. Overcoming what we perceive as shortcomings brings us positive psychological benefits, which is why "risk recreation" and dangerous sports are becoming increasingly popular. Participating in satisfying hobbies helps us to receive what psychologists call "self-actualization." Extreme sports like parachute jumping, white-water rafting, and mountain climbing provide extra benefits because they encourage us to take risks. In fact, they give us a little thrill from doing so. Push yourself on your weak points, but also try things like jumping from a high diving board, practicing on a sports center climbing wall, or trying a low rappel. You can work your way up, and if you conquer your fears you'll become more inclined to sensation seeking. Phew! Your partner had better watch out!

Are you unduly worried about getting too sweaty or soiling the sheets during sex? Turn to IDEA 51, *Sheer filth.*

Try another idea...

"The musician who never gets past technique never really plays music. Similarly, the lover who thinks primarily about technique never really makes love."
KIM CATTRALL and MARK LEVINSON, *Satisfaction*

Defining idea...

How did it go?

Q **Aren't men more prone to indulging in risky behavior?**

A *Yes. The gene SRY, sometimes called the "gene for maleness," switches on other genes that create male traits. This includes a tendency to take greater risks, which is why men have a shorter average lifespan than women. In* Nature via Nurture, *Matt Ridley quotes Randolph Nesse: "The average rate of violent death among men was higher in hunter-gatherer societies than it was in war-torn twentieth-century Germany." Indulging in a little risky behavior is good, but too much can be fatal!*

Q **Isn't it easier to take stuff like alcohol and drugs as a fail-safe way to get over inhibitions?**

A *Yes, as a short-term solution. As sex really originates in the mind, finding a way to confront any guilt or fears we're experiencing is crucial. There's no denying there are wonderful drugs that do the job for you and alcohol is the classic de-inhibitor; however, when these wear off you may end up feeling more guilty/uncomfortable in your normal state. This makes it more likely you'll turn to them again as a crutch: a vicious circle situation. It's also a plus if you can remember the high points of any sexual experience!*

34

Pandora's box

Porn is not just *Playboy*. A glimpse of the weird and wonderful world of pornography. If you're astounded at what turns others on, have you explored all your erotic possibilities?

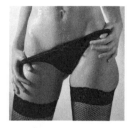

What's promoted as sexy is invariably found in mainstream porn, but this is not what actually turns on every man, or you. Do you dare to discover something different?

Porn often makes us feel insecure, simply because our bodies don't look like the perfect poses on show in the likes of *Playboy* and *Hustler*. A friend of mine, Kristina Etchison, was production manager on over twenty porn magazines at Larry Flynt Publications and told me how they got the girls to thrust their breasts out "because it makes you look thinner" and how every inch of skin is ruthlessly Photoshopped for a flawless effect. Girls often have special body makeup, and might have had labioplasty to even things up—so even naked they're not "natural."

However, there are magazines and websites that cater to every fantasy and predilection; some get off on fetishizing part of the body, such as *Legs,* or prefer to see women partially clad, as in *Panty Play*. It might surprise you to know that some

Here's an idea for you... **Arrange a party with your girlfriends. Along with the bottles of wine, ask everyone to bring some porn they find stimulating. By the end of the night you should have had a laugh and discovered some tantalizing stuff.**

men seek hairy, large, or "mature" women as a sexual preference and there are numerous magazines that cater to this. In the West, older and plumper female images are often presented in a tasteless, "nasty sex" way. This is a world away from the ideology of most black magazines, which operate in a cultural norm where big really is beautiful. *Belle's* target audience is "confident full-figured women" and its sister magazine *Love and Lingerie* contains stunning photographs of large women that make you realize that, hey, these women do look amazing: gorgeous underwear isn't just for those who are a size six.

Of course, there are adult magazines aimed at women, too; *Scarlet, For Women,* and *Playgirl* cover all aspects of erotica and feature male pinups; www.forthegirls.com is an erotica site with photos specially chosen for women. Lesbian magazines like *Diva* and *Curve* present female sexuality in an alternative way and often have more interesting articles. If you prefer a good read, try the *Erotic Review Forum,* www.erotica-readers.com, or my favorite, www.nerve.com, which was set up because "sex is beautiful and absurd, remarkably fun and reliably trauma-inducing." Sex content doesn't have to appeal to the lowest common denominator. Larry

Defining idea... **"Pornography is a matter of geography."**
JOHN PATRICK, playwright

Flynt Publications experimented with the now defunct *Rage* magazine, which combined searing political content and sexy spreads with sardonic captions for the male reader: "Why don't you put it back in your pants, zip up, and go get a 'real' girl? Your woman may not look this good, but at least she's not a paper doll who only lives in fantasy."

If perusing porn inspires you, why not make your own? Check out IDEA 39, _Girls on film_.

Try another idea...

Fetish magazines tend to be high quality and glossy, and less overtly in-your-face sexual. The most glamorous is _Marquis_, which features beautiful fetish fashion; _Skin Two_ contains more articles around the scene, and _Secret_ is focused on bondage. We're still just scratching the surface but this should give you an idea of the competing ideals for what constitutes "sexy" and what makes you hot.

Your aim in perusing adult magazines, websites, and books is to remap your own sexual boundaries. What turns you on and which sexual ideologies do you identify with? Try to avoid an "us versus them" approach. It doesn't matter if you don't look like Jenna Jameson because there's a whole counterculture of porn that rejects the blonde, big-breasted ideal, and we all fit someone's fantasy. The most important thing is to be happy being you. In _The Beauty Myth_ Naomi Wolf says, "in terms of how we feel about ourselves _physically_, we may actually be worse off than our unliberated grandmothers." Remember, variety is the spice of life.

How did
it go?

Q   Doesn't pornography exploit women?

A   *This issue has been hotly debated by feminists, but Sarah Jane Hamilton, former porn star turned director, says that actresses profit much more from porn than actors: "A top woman can command $10,000 a movie, a top male gets $500 a day." The adult industry is now one that creates franchises out of its female brands, a far cry from the furtive business it once was. Anne McClintock also defends S&M pornography in an article in* Dirty Looks: Women, Pornography, Power. *She says, "it is also commonly thought that men who pay for commercial S&M pay to indulge in the sadistic abuse of women. Yet the testimony of dominatrixes reveals precisely the opposite. By far the most common service paid for by men in heterosexual S&M is the extravagant display of submission."*

Q   Why do we need pornography anyway?

A   *Pornography has always been at the forefront of every new technology; it heralded the beginning of film and helped to popularize the introduction of video machines and the Internet. A third of all Internet searches involve some form of pornography, and 40 percent of those surfers are estimated to be women. The number of American couples seeking porno rentals has increased. Laura Kipness says, "Perhaps the abundance of pornography simply resonates with a primary desire for plenitude, for pleasure without social limits." The French writer Alain Robbe-Grillet insists it's necessary: "An adult needs pornography as a child needs fairy tales."*

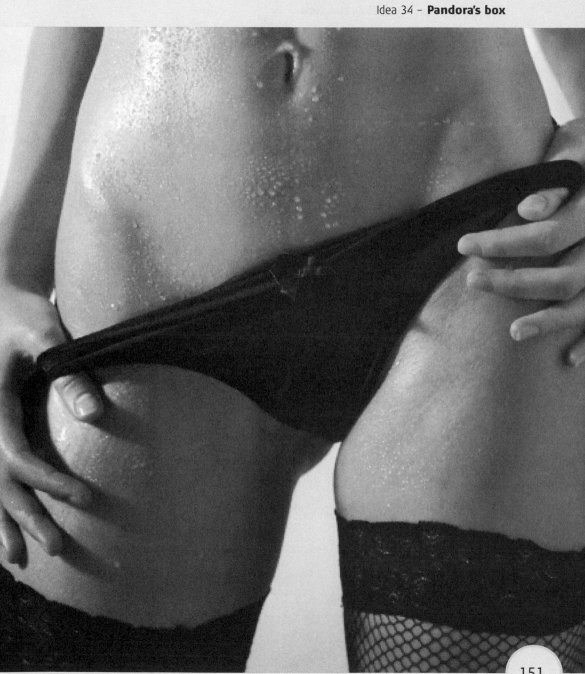

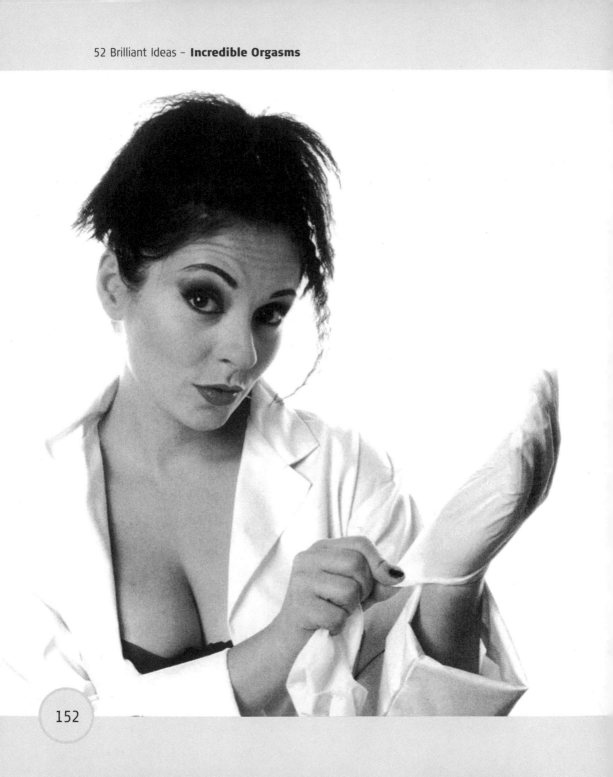

35

Beyond the beyond

The road to excess leads to the palace of wisdom. Tips for the sexually adventurous (not for the fainthearted).

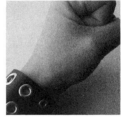

Advanced sex play makes use of new techniques. Fisting or handballing is popular among lesbian couples and offers a completely different approach to penetration.

You might be surprised to know that what you do in the bedroom is influenced by what professional performers get up to in porn. Sex has fashions, and porn leads the way on what we think is hot, sexy, and funky. In the '70s and '80s porn made oral sex mainstream. In the '90s anal sex became a must-do, and now female performers are going one further and doing stuff like double anal penetration. At the same time porn has become more visible so if you want to have wild sex like Jenna Jameson, here are some tips to help you along.

For advanced play you need new techniques. For example, instead of just penetration, you might want to experiment with fisting, which is popular in the lesbian community. Patrick Califia says in *Sensuous Magic*, "Contrary to what the name of this technique would lead you to believe, you do not make a fist and then

Here's an idea for you...

If fisting is not for you, make up your own "slave" contract and both sign it. You can find a sample one on www.houseofdesade.org, and use this as the basis to create your own. You don't have to do S&M, you can use it to stipulate sexual rights and housework negotiation. Try it for a limited period and see if it increases your fun quota.

somehow wedge it into the vagina." If you're new to it, get your partner to do it for you. He must be patient (fisting can take up to an hour) and slow, and learn to work with how much your vagina muscles can take. Beforehand he should wash his hands (his nails must be trimmed) and remove his watch. Wearing a latex glove is optional.

Start by lubricating with a water-based lube and playing around with one finger, adding others one at a time. You have to be incredibly horny to be able to enjoy this. Using lots of stimulation and lube, get him to play with you and slowly add more fingers. See how far you can go. If he can insert four fingers, you're nearly there and it's just a question of him squashing his fingers together and twisting his hand to go further in. If it becomes uncomfortable, take some of the fingers out or stop altogether. A diagonal route is the best way to get the whole hand in.

Defining idea...

"The only unnatural sex act is that which you cannot perform."
DR. ALFRED KINSEY

Some women describe being fisted as the ultimate orgasm and when this happens, your muscles might clench so much they push his hand out. He has to go with the flow, but must never take his hand out quickly—it can take as long to get out as it took to get in, so this is not an activity to do in the five minutes before bedtime. If the vaginal opening forms what Califia describes as a "vacuum seal" around his wrist, get him to insert a finger to break "the seal."

If you enjoy this, Emily Dubberley recommends self-fisting in *Brief Encounters*. It's not as easy doing it yourself as having it done for you, but it gives you a chance to experiment. This time it's you masturbating yourself and slowly sliding in more fingers. Dubberley says, "Once you get to the knuckles, twist your hand more to get it inside you. The angle is pretty tricky, so you may need your other hand to help ease your fist inside yourself." The difficult bit is getting the fist in (it's the biggest part) but once it's in there it gets easier.

The advantage of fisting is that it makes your pleasure the focus of the sexual experience and requires your partner/you to spend a long time achieving it, things that women don't demand enough. According to Susie Bright at susiebright.com women who took part in her sex surveys are having fewer orgasms and Bright says, "Young women are incredibly preoccupied with whether they are pleasing their man, rather than being pleased themselves with sex." Fisting is not for everyone, but some say it's the ultimate female indulgence.

If you want to try some new things out but lack confidence, mentally prepare yourself first with IDEA 33, *Let yourself go.*

 Try another idea...

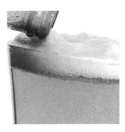

"I hate to advocate drugs, alcohol, violence, or insanity to anyone, but they've always worked for me."
HUNTER S. THOMPSON

Defining idea...

How did
it go?

Q   Isn't this a bit extreme for the average woman?

A   *Women are designed for a much more extreme activity—giving birth. It could be that fisting isn't for you, but getting your partner to play around with how many fingers he can insert could make for great, prolonged foreplay. Think of it as a goal that gives you an excuse to get pleasured more; whether he gets all his fingers in or not is not really the issue. For a more in-depth guide to this subject see* A Hand in the Bush: The Fine Art of Vaginal Fisting *by Deborah Addington.*

Q   Are there any medical side effects?

A   *You can encounter medical problems with almost any activity. Fisting is no exception. Emily Dubberley warns, "Fisting can damage nerves in the bladder, G-spot, urethral sphincter, and cervix through abrasion or over-stretching. It can also encourage cystitis . . ." The key is to do it slowly and to stop at once if it feels painful. You'll soon learn to know what you can and can't take. The point of any extreme activity, whether it's climbing Mount Everest or riding a bucking bronco, is that it has that element of danger. Anyway, in the S&M community what's regarded as extreme is stuff like playing with fire, bone scratching, and hanging from flesh hooks. So, relatively, fisting is not that far out!*

36

Mix it up

Although you've tried half the *Kama Sutra*, you know what you like. Even if it works for you, doing the same thing, around the same time, gets old.

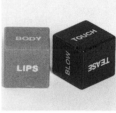

Remember the gold-covered women in "Goldfinger"? Here's how to paint and play with each other to your heart's content. It's silly but it works wonders.

It's easy to get stuck in a rut. In fact, psychologists J. D. Watt and J. E. Ewing say sexual boredom may be the most destructive problem for couples. In reality, lack of desire is not really about the sex, but a state of general boredom that expresses itself most poignantly in the bedroom. Although arousal feels biological, it's actually all in the mind. The trick is to feel more upbeat generally and to spend more time with other people. A 2001 study on boredom proneness found that people who get bored quickly were more likely to suffer from loneliness and engage in solitary sexual practices. Having a rowdy dinner party is the perfect way to start that warm feeling of contentment for the weekend. My friends and I had a hilarious time trying out some of the more adventurous sexual positions (fully clothed) illustrated in various sex books! Do fun things and enjoy yourself and you'll get to your sexual activities in the right frame of mind.

Here's an idea for you...

If you're not that concerned about new underwear or sex toys, why not try some liquid latex? You can buy it and simply paint it on your body. It's best to shave before applying it (then it's easier to remove), and you can use it to create temporary underwear. Three coats are recommended and each takes around ten minutes to dry. After use, simply peel it off. Imagine the fun you could have decorating each other's bodies!

Defining idea...

"Not everything that is faced can be changed; but nothing can be changed until it is faced."
JAMES BALDWIN

Rather than concentrating on hot new techniques, being more playful in the bedroom works wonders. For instance, you could play Twister naked or stage a food fight: anything to get you having fun together. You can try strip poker or spin the bottle. Sites like www.mypleasure.com are teeming with erotic games to play on a rainy day. A game like Nookii is designed specifically for couples and helps to initiate foreplay and daring sexual moves. Players move around each other's bodies rather than a game board with instructions like: "Moisten my nipples, then, with a gentle pinch, trigger their pertness." For a gentle introduction to playing at S&M, the Sensual Sweet Surrender game gives you rules and props such as a blindfold, feather, rubber tickler, and flavored massage oil. Although it's a bonus if you get turned on by these activities, don't be afraid just to play around.

Another bonus of play is that it's a chance to freely experience each other's naked bodies. If you feel more comfortable being fresh out of the shower, then do this first. Maybe you need to refresh your tan or get a pedicure; do what you need to get rid of any inhibitions. Then you can try stuff to decorate and lick off the body. Feel free to get out a sieve and be creative with cocoa and icing sugar. Can you decorate someone's breasts neatly with strawberry sauce?

Alternatively, you can get professional and play with the Body Talk Tattoo Set, which contains stencils, brushes, and chocolate frosting with commands that you can temporarily paint onto the body. And then there's lick-off body gel and body finger paints for you to have fun with. Regular makeup can also be used on body parts; use lip and eye liners to write messages. Another fun game is to appliqué small shells, sequins, sweets, whatever, onto people's bodies using tepid wax. It's a laugh and it gets the fun back. And you need this sense of fun if you want to try out specifically sexual things like new positions, erogenous zones, or sex toys.

When we talk about changing, most people imagine a radical change, but taking small steps is enough. Be prepared to try on each other's underwear or roll around in chocolate sauce and you're pretty much road-tested for anything!

Once you're comfortable having a laugh doing silly stuff, it's easier to move on to trying out new sex toys: see IDEA 13, *Toys R no fuss.*

Try another idea...

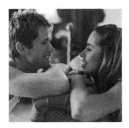

"Marriage must incessantly be content with a monster that devours everything: familiarity."
HONORÉ DE BALZAC

Defining idea...

159

How did
it go?

Q   My partner is too inhibited to do stuff like this. What can I do?

A   *Easy—just use positive reinforcement. You know when you take a dog for a walk and give it treats to persuade it to behave in a certain way? Men are no different. Even when you make small changes, praise him, encouraging him to continue. If he does something to please you then indulge him in something he enjoys. Avoid making sweeping changes; in the end you get further taking it slow and steady. Find ways to make him laugh and you're halfway there.*

Q   Isn't this all a bit childish?

A   *Yes, but that's the effect we're striving for. Our ability to play games is crucial to our inner life of erotic fantasy and to give us confidence to try new things. Psychologist Dr. Michael Bader says in his book* Arousal: The Secret Logic of Sexual Fantasies, *"The capacity to sustain the tension between imagination and reality is central to our ability to play, to pretend that something is real while knowing that it is invented, to play games with rules that we create and then treat it as if they were an immutable part of the outside world . . ." Life itself is like playing a spectacularly long game of* Monopoly. *Treat sex with a bit of childishness—go on, enjoy yourself!*

37

Eyes wide shut

For a different buzz, try cutting off one of the senses—it can intensify the others. Just when you thought you'd tried it all, discover the sublime art of sensory deprivation.

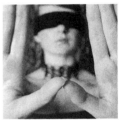

If you think blindfolds are just for a bit of kink, think again. A simple blindfold can give you hours of fun, heighten your erotic potential, and even doubles as a party game.

Our senses are more complex and individual than we realized. Although it's generally accepted that we have five senses, in 2005 the *New Scientist* published an article that claimed we have up to twenty-one. This is because we have more receptors that interpret each sense: with sight, for instance, the way we see colors is different from the way we perceive shade. Sight is particularly important because like other primates we've swapped a good sense of smell for full color vision. If you blindfold someone it has more of an effect than, say, changing their sense of taste. It's also one of the easiest senses to block and you can use things like a pair of tights, a scarf, or even bandages under sunglasses to achieve it.

Although almost anything can be used as a blindfold, try to use something appropriate. The anonymous author of www.geocities.com/Hollywood/Theater/7699

Here's an idea for you...

For the ultimate in sensory deprivation, try a floatation tank experience. It's a way of getting the deepest relaxation possible, and one hour of floating is equivalent to four hours of sleep. Search online to find somewhere you and your partner can book adjoining rooms and I'll leave it up to you what happens afterward . . .

says, "Choose a blindfold that fits the occasion. Strike a balance between blocking out light, looks, and comfort." He advises using a double knot to prevent the blindfold from slipping, although if your partner is lying down you can use a single knot in a cotton scarf, which is more comfortable. You can experiment with different colored cloth, wet blindfolds, or textures, such as playdough wrapped in plastic. Alternatively, professional leather-lined blindfolds are sold in most sex shops and are inexpensive. Going one step further, you can use a blindfold and a hood, and even disposable plastic earplugs to block out two senses in one go.

The person being blindfolded is going to experience more sensory sensitivity in the other areas so even mundane activities can take on a whole new meaning. You could get someone, for instance, to try eating dinner blindfold, or taking a (supervised) bath and let them experience their skin with their super-heightened sense of hearing and touch. Now's the time to experiment with erotic audio CDs in the bedroom: try the Herotica series edited by Marcy Sheiner—this range of women-only audio stories is perfect for getting you turned on. Good Vibrations also sells apt mood music, Cyberorgasm CDs that give you orgasms, and gasps in surround-sound. Another strategy is for the other person to change the furniture in the room in advance and to frequently move about to disorient the blindfolded one. If you've got the blindfold on him, wear your highest heels—the sound of you walking around in them becomes exotic.

Complement physical sensory deprivation with mental challenges. See IDEA 20, *Mind games*.

Try another idea…

In this state you can really appreciate erotic massage, being fed a range of raw fruits, or being kissed by someone who alternates between drinking something hot and cold. It's all about surprise and anticipation and you can use this to prolong your foreplay. Sensory deprivation technique is especially good for couples who have gotten used to each other a bit too much and need something new. When you're feeling helpless, the introduction of ice-cube play feels out of this world. Or if he's blindfolded you can pretend to be two women and role-play any fantasy you care to enjoy. You can use different voices, clothes, and sexual moves on him and pretend to be someone else.

You can take this play as far as you like (some dominatrixes specialize in cutting off all the senses one by one using gags, hoods, earplugs, menthol vapor rub—and then bringing them back). Alternatively you can use the blindfold to give someone a surprise; it's great when you want to heighten the suspense for present giving or whisk someone away to an exotic location. It's easy, safe, and fun—you're only limited by your imagination.

"Each of us lives in our own sensory world forged by memory, experience and individual physiology."
HESTON BLUMENTHAL, chef

Defining idea…

How did it go?

Q   **Aren't blindfolds a bit boring?**

A   *They're just a simple tool. What you do with them can turn your play into something exciting, scary, or relaxing. You can play lots of games and role-play using these and it doesn't have to be sexual. (Remember those party games you did as a kid that use blindfolds?) Check out the largest list of blindfold games on the web for a truly mind-opening selection of things to do.*

Q   **Sorry, I can't take this seriously. Is this just kids' stuff or is it getting into wacko territory?**

A   *It's true that sensory deprivation has its dark side, and kidnappers and interrogators make use of it to disorient their victims. To keep your play safe, never go to sleep with a blindfold on as it can slip down and potentially strangle you in the night. If you are hooded or gagged, use a marble that you can drop as the equivalent of a safe word. While blindfolds are great for party games of all ages, don't underestimate your sensory abilities. After doing a nude skydive, NASA flight surgeon Angus Rupert produced the world's first tactile flight suit; our reflexes for touch are faster than those using sight, and if you plug this suit in to the cockpit you can fly blindfold. Hardly just kids' stuff!*

164

38

Finding it

Sometimes staying at home is not where it's at. Meet like-minded people; try visiting an alternative club, sauna, or workshop. If that feels like too much, visit a sex shop.

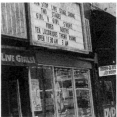

If your sex drive is down in the doldrums, pep it up by doing something new, different, or sensual. Don't get stuck in a rut; get out of the house and go.

You already know the biggest sexual organ is your brain and that negative self-image is the quickest way to erode desire. In a recent survey, 90 percent of women felt more depressed after seeing pictures of impossibly glamorous women. To counter this, try going to a sauna where you'll actually get to see real women naked: young, old, fat, and everything in between—the experience is normalizing. Yep, it's OK not to look like Kate Moss. Learn to feel more at ease sitting in your own skin and pamper yourself a little. Even if you feel shy at first (try a woman-only session if you're particularly bothered), you'll wonder what all the fuss was about ten minutes later once you're naked. Nonsexual nudity makes you freer, puts you in touch with yourself, and helps lose those inhibitions. It's physically good for your body, too— saunas improve circulation and relieve a sluggish digestive system. Even though a

Promise yourself that next weekend you will go to a new club or spa. Dare yourself to enter a new erotic territory; for example, a gay or transvestite hangout where you can buzz off an alternative vibe. Search online for the right location, and use the opportunity to check out some web forums on the local scene and chat to a few people beforehand.

sauna is a nonerotic experience for most of us, it will stimulate you mentally and physically, an ideal step to open you up to erotic possibilities.

Other delights to indulge in include a full body massage. Our bodies respond positively to touch regardless of whether this is erotic or not, and a relaxed body is primed for better orgasms. If letting a stranger work his hands all over you is too much, try having a reflexology session instead; only your feet are massaged but these have reflexes that correspond to every part of the body. Mmm, feel good?

Once you've shed some of your inhibitions, you're ready to paint the town red. Check local listings for details of clubs, events, and workshops—and why not something alternative? Are you prepared to go to an exhibition of nudes? It's not much of a step, then, to go to a safe sex workshop or an erotic writing class; writers like Mitzi Szereto teach erotic writing at locations all over the world.

"If you don't risk anything you risk even more."
ERICA JONG author

You could also try going to different clubs. Many straight women feel at home in a gay club where any interaction is free from the "meat-market" mentality of regular clubs. Being around others who are sexually confident rubs off and you should aim to go home feeling fabulous. You might even want to try a fetish club. Normally there is a dress code (leather, latex, uniform) but once you're inside you'll find that there's plenty to watch without having to be a "player." Many love the theatrical drama of dressing up and being on show—it's not quite the hard-core,

If you believe that feeling sexy is only for the young and beautiful, read IDEA 4, *The beautiful and the bad*, to see what kind of angst celebrities actually harbor.

Try another idea...

wall-to-wall gangbang the popular press makes out. You don't have to do anything sexual, but again it's a chance to open up and find something new to turn you on—and you'll be telling your friends all about it for weeks afterward.

If you have a particular fetish or interest (such as leather, bondage, naturism) hook up with like-minded people. You can generally find these online or in listing magazines like *Time Out*. It's a chance to swap ideas, pick up tips, and mingle with potential partners all at the same time. Most groups offer a whirl of social events and give you the opportunity to indulge in your passions. Elizabeth Thorne says a fun way to become active in the scene is to volunteer to help with events: "You have a safe and directed way to interact with people."

If the very thought of going to a fetish club leaves you cold, visit a sex shop. Many are women-friendly, well-lit, and offer a discreet, professional service. When I persuaded a friend to go to one, she was pleasantly surprised. Do anything, but do something!

"If I had to live my life again, I'd make the same mistakes, only sooner."
TALLULAH BANKHEAD

Defining idea...

How did it go?

Q   I never have orgasms. How can going out gallivanting help me in the bedroom?

A   *There are lots of theories on why women are anorgasmic (can't come). Sex therapist Peg Burr suggests it's related to feeling out of control. On Queendom.com Burr says, "Orgasm requires becoming vulnerable and open. This openness is based on an intact sense of self which does not feel threatened (engulfed, or overpowered) by sexual union. Persons who are rigid and/or controlling have great difficulty allowing themselves to be vulnerable and completely orgasmically responsive with another person . . ." Bearing all that in mind, any activity which you do voluntarily should help to prevent the nagging feeling of being out of control. Take small, slow steps, be relaxed in every situation.*

Q   I don't like the thought of being naked in a sauna or going skimpily dressed to a club, although I'm interested in going to these places . . . What now?

A   *It's a bit like that first plunge into a cold swimming pool. Get it over and done with as quickly as possible. In countries like Germany nakedness is compulsory in saunas, but you can still hold a towel around you and cover up your bits (I do, as a blushing expat). In some places a swimsuit is OK. Most women sit with their arms partially covering their breasts, so you can't see much anyway. As regards clubs, the good thing about fetish wear is that materials like latex, rubber, and Lycra allow you to be covered head to toe while revealing every curve.*

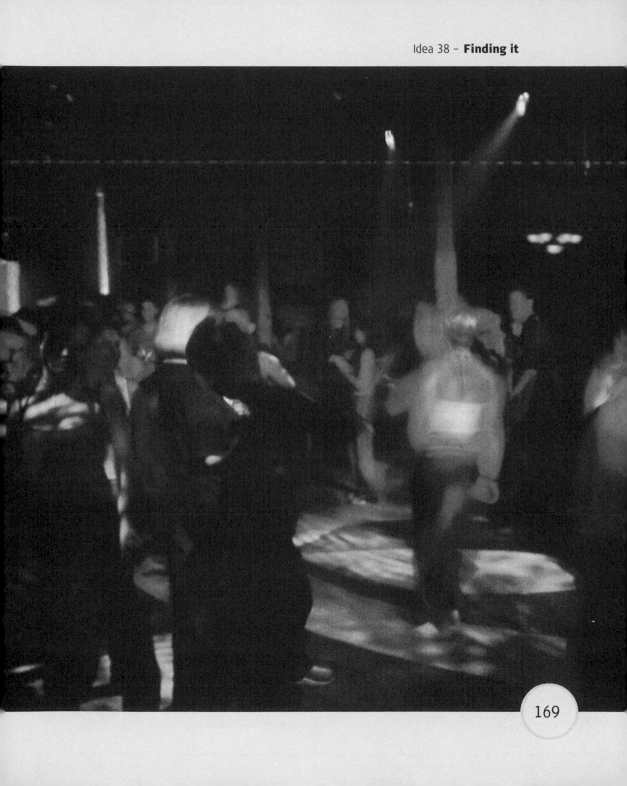

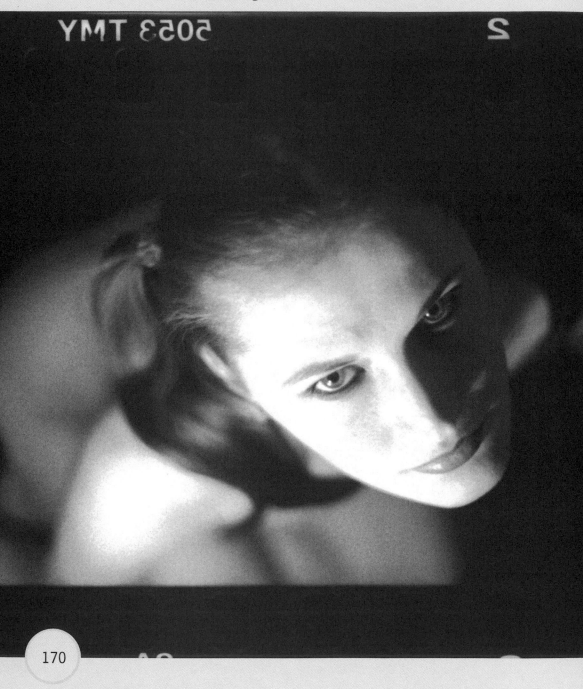

39

Girls on film

Find ways to immortalize your other life—the one devoted to passion. Anything from taking photos to making your own home movie can be an incentive to keep the passion flowing.

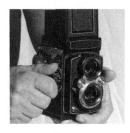

You need a lot of trust to photograph or film each other nude doing rude things, but it can build intimacy, spice up your love life, and give you a few visual tips.

Perhaps seeing yourself, nude and aroused, or in situ with your lover, could give you more of an insight into your relationship and yourself. We live in a world saturated with sexual images, but we probably don't know what we look like in our most intimate moments. After all, you have photographs of all those other special occasions—graduating from high school or college, your twenty-first birthday, celebration dinners, but next to nothing about sexual milestones that are seared forever in your brain. Capturing some of your sex life on tape helps to make it seem more real, and a lot of it is going on; video cameras now appear in the top twenty list of sex toys.

Here's an idea for you... **If you're anxious about having photos/videos hanging around, get your lover to draw you in the nude like they do in art class. Of course, he can dictate any poses he thinks fit, and they'll probably be far raunchier than the standard poses students work with.**

Begin by spending time just looking at yourself naked in front of a full-length mirror. What parts of yourself do you most like and dislike? No woman is 100 percent happy with all parts of her body (Cameron Diaz apparently doesn't like her butt), but embrace all of it. Rub body lotion or massage oil all over to give yourself a sexy sheen and practice a few poses. Go on, push out your breasts and make your back taller, pulling in your tummy. Look around from the back, sit on a chair with your legs astride, try anything you like and see how it feels.

Perhaps you'll feel more comfortable photographing yourself in private first. This exercise is a great excuse to buy something sexy, and remember the easiest way to make a naked body look better is to get an even tan and to regularly moisturize all over, so do the preparation work. You can set up a video camera and leave it running while you practice walking, undressing, posing, or even masturbating. Play it back to yourself later and note how you moved and how any clothes you wore suited you. This is a great opportunity to parade around in those sexy items lurking at the back of the drawer. You could also use the photo function on your mobile phone to snap all kinds of strange positions down there, or set up a regular camera to go off at timed intervals. You'll probably find you look totally different from how you imagined; edit the film or photos, keeping the ones that are the most flattering.

Defining idea... *"When pornography sneezes, pop culture catches cold."*
IRVINE WELSH

Take a good look at your vagina. Do your vaginal lips change when you're aroused? Are there any visual markers like swelling or going redder that your lover can pick up on? Use this exercise to lose some inhibitions, and try out any sex toys you have. If you're happy with the results you could always leave the tape around for your lover to "accidentally" find!

For depilation tips and that "porn star" look, see IDEA 28, A hairy situation

Try another idea...

If you want to immortalize each other together, lay down some ground rules first. In an online article Rodney Chester warns, "Making a porn video is just one step. What to do with it is another problem." It could be that one of you keeps it in a safe place, or that you don masks for the filming, or only shoot nonidentifiable body parts. We all know what happens when homemade porn leaks out from the scandals around the Pamela Anderson and Paris Hilton tapes.

Now you're ready to experiment. Perhaps you're choreographing everything around a narrative—like a sexy nurse and a sick patient. Take the chance to flesh out your fantasies. Later you can analyze your foreplay strategies and put a voice to the images, telling your lover what things turned you on the most. It's a chance to learn something and develop trust, and it might turn you on: it's really the perfect rainy day activity!

Defining idea...

"I have no regrets about keeping our sex off-camera. But I also don't have any evidence that I was once a recklessly drunk, stupid, skinny, daring, bold young woman . . ."
LISA GABRIELE, journalist

How did
it go?

Q   Isn't DIY porn a bit seedy?

A   *It depends on how you film it. You don't have to shoot rude areas at all (and in fact, unless you have a half-decent cameraman in with you, you're simply not going to get classic genital close-ups, everything will be in long shot when you are filmed together). Photographs of laughing and smiling can equally be alluring, as the photographer Whitney Lawson says: "Photographing lust is easy. Trying to photograph love, on the other hand, is like trying to pin a wave on the sand . . ."*

Q   Why is amateur porn so popular right now?

A   *The technology is cheap and accessible; it's also a kind of craze according to novelist Irvine Welsh: "Everyone seems to be involved in sex clubs now in Edinburgh. People go to a pub, then they all go back to each others' houses, shag each other senseless and get it on the DVD. It's become a social thing, like a dinner party." Google cofounder Larry Page announced in 2005 that the company wanted the public to send in homemade videos, including DIY porn. Although publicly they need the tapes to test their prototype video search software, it seems to have a commercial value. We now have "Gonzo porn" that is designed to look amateurish because a lot of traditional porn looks too clichéd. Amateur sex has become synonymous with "real" sex.*

40

Love at first sight

Are you predestined to fall in love? Or perhaps you're bonkers about a certain type? Delving into the mysterious properties of love . . .

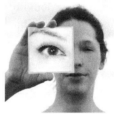

Songwriters, painters, writers, and our own experiences tell us that love is real. But what is it really and how do we fall in love?

Although sexual diversity is all the rage, monogamy is still the most common form of bonding for humans. We are the only species (apart from the bonobo chimpanzee) that has sex face-to-face and often feels bound to a particular individual, even when there are richer, more attractive pickings elsewhere. Sometimes we're mystified by why X is the "true love" of Y; for most of us it was a revelation to find Prince Charles loved Camilla Parker Bowles when he was married to one of the most beautiful women in the world—Diana. Suzi Malin in *Love at First Sight* thinks Camilla is an example of prima copulism: "an attachment based on a visual resemblance to a person's first bond." Although this is often a mother or a sister, in this case Camilla looks uncannily like Mabel Anderson, Charles's first nanny.

Another "visual love category" is harmonism, where two people's faces are not the same shape but appear in the same proportions. To see if you have this trait with a

Here's an idea for you...

Take photographs of you and your partner where you are looking in the same direction. If you have a computer, scan in the two images and scale them so they are the same size, or use a photocopier. Draw a horizontal line above the upper eyelids and another one through the center of the mouths to see if you have harmonism (where your faces are in the same proportions). Fold the images in half and match both sides of your faces together to see if you have a perfect match.

lover, cut two photographs in half (try to photocopy or scan them to roughly the same size first). Look at the length of the nose and compare this to the gap between the forehead and the nose, and the distance between the mouth and the nose. Malin cites Hugh Grant and Liz Hurley as a classic example of two people who share harmonist elements; their basic face shapes are in proportion.

The final visual category to look for is echoism, where couples actually physically resemble each other. Look at the line of the eye, lip, and eyebrow: if they mirror each other, like David and Victoria Beckham, then you've got a strong couple because they share basic similarities. (Even animals choose mates that are similar to themselves.) It's easy to spot this on two photos lying side by side that have been taken from the same angle.

Defining idea...

"The meeting of two personalities is like the contact of two chemical substances: if there is any reaction, both are transformed."
CARL JUNG

There are a number of other factors that can trigger infatuation. We each possess an "odor print" as unique as our fingerprint and we recognize the smells of people long after we've forgotten what they look like because our sense of smell is part of the limbic system, which is connected to long-term memory. Does your favorite lover's smell remind you of something else?

If you're a bad-boy magnet, check out IDEA 44, *The rake*, for the low-down on why you're attracted to these types.

Try another idea...

Other factors could be what the psychologist John Money calls your "love map," an image of what you think is thrilling and sexy that is a composite of all the images and thoughts that you've ever assembled to create your "ideal lover." We unconsciously pick up on the actors in TV shows, characters in books, our schoolmates and form an ideal by the age of six! This is a bit difficult to check, but go back through your old stuff; can you make a connection?

Sometimes having a challenge makes us more determined: psychologist Dorothy Tennov did a survey of 800 people about falling in love and found that having an obstacle only inflames the passion, but she also concluded that you only fall in love when you are ready for it. As Helen E. Fisher concludes in *The Anatomy of Love*, "It is this constellation of factors appearing *all* at once—including timing, barriers, mystery, similarities, a matched love map, even the right smells—that make you susceptible to falling in love." Look for the signs and don't be surprised at the crazy reasons why you are mad about someone.

"This madness, this limerance, this attraction, this infatuation, this ecstasy so regularly ignored by scientists, must be a universal human trait."
HELEN E. FISHER, author

Defining idea...

How did it go?

Q Aren't echoism and harmonism a bit far-fetched?

A No. According to anthropologists we prefer to mate with those who have similar characteristics because there's less chance of genetic mutation. Helen E. Fisher says in Anatomy of Love, *"Likes tend to marry likes— individuals of the same ethnic groups, with similar physical traits and levels of education, what anthropologists call positive assertive mating." According to Plato, God cut our ancestors in half for our sins and we're still trying to reunite!*

Q Isn't love actually a chemical reaction?

A Yes, it is. When you're attracted to someone your brain releases phenylethylamine, or PEA, which is mildly hallucinogenic, as well as the chemical dopamine, which gives you a feeling of well-being. After the initial attraction, the hormone oxytocin takes over, which creates a feeling of closeness, just like the bond between a woman and her newborn baby. In The Science of Love, *Anthony Walsh says, "PEA is a revved-up feeling, like the one cocaine produces. It is the Bon Jovi of hormones. Oxytocin is more relaxed. It is what helps us to stay together. Think of it as Beethoven." No wonder love is such a good feeling!*

41

Relationships revisited

**Are you getting the full potential out of your partner?
Couples can get sloppy so put the *oomph* back into your
sex life. And that means both of you!**

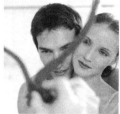

In a long-term relationship the way you
relate in everyday life affects your sexual
chemistry, so give each other a bit of respect.

These days women have more career and lifestyle opportunities, but it's difficult to
balance everything and to determine who does what in the division of labor at
home. Sadly, women are still doing more housework than their male partners and
the arrival of children only makes the situation worse. Melissa Benn writes that the
new type of woman emerging in surveys is "not so much having it all as doing it all"
and their male partners are so absent that "their partners may as well be single
parents." In *Wifework: What Marriage Really Means for Women* Susan Maushart says,
"Childless marriages are 'equaler.' Parenting really does force people—often against
their conscious wills—back into traditional grooves." To top it off, we're also
working longer and harder. Madeleine Bunting points out that US corporations are
getting more working hours per family: "In 1970, it took one parent to pay for a
lifestyle that in 2000 takes two."

Here's an idea for you... **Remember the things you did in the first months of your relationship in a whirl of romance? Go back to that restaurant where you first held hands and rent films you saw together at the theater. Revisiting your past will reinforce your bond together and hopefully this enthusiasm will spill over into the bedroom.**

Not surprisingly, stress and overwork take their toll on relationships, and it's easy to take each other for granted. It's important to talk regularly; even chatting about apparently trivial things, like what happened at work about the broken coffee machine, shows that you both care and are interested in what the other is doing. The Equality in Marriage Institute says poor communication is the most common complaint of couples seeking counseling. When we're in a hurry, taking the time to have half an hour's chat may be the first thing that's sacrificed, but repeatedly ignoring your partner's needs will only build up problems later on—and one of the first things to be affected is your love life. Make time to talk, and kick back with each other if you have issues: it's better to hash them out than ignore them. Of course, talking isn't the same as communicating. Each individual has her own attitudes about what is normal or acceptable, which can put you at cross-purposes. Choosing a good time to bring difficult things up is also an art in itself; it's obviously better for him to avoid the subject of your unruly office if you have a conference presentation deadline looming.

Of course, for couples in trouble there is never a good time, because underlying resentment has built up. Steer clear of this by learning to talk through issues together. You don't win an argument if you've browbeaten someone into submission, so discuss solutions and compromises instead. Remain positive and ensure your body language doesn't betray what you're really thinking. Only 7 percent of emotional meaning is verbal: in other words, if you have a heated discussion curled up together on the sofa, it's going to be a lot harder for one of you to take it badly.

If you're super busy, check out **IDEA 21, *Compromise positions*,** for quick sex tips to keep your love life on the boil.

A particular problem for women is how their lifestyle fits in with feminist ideals of gender equality when their own relationship might fall somewhat short of an ideal partnership. A recent survey found that 55 percent of couples with children argue over cleaning and suggested it would be better for men to do some work around the house instead of buying traditional gifts for Valentine's Day. Dr. Eustace Chesser says in *Woman and Love* that women are biologically programmed to see intercourse not as a single sex act but as a series of moments to be celebrated; everything that your partner does in the day leading up to intercourse can affect your mood and perception of the physical act. It's beautifully simple: if you and your partner respect and help each other, your sex life is more likely to be passionate and full-bodied.

"What counts in making a happy marriage is not so much how compatible you are, but how you deal with incompatibility."
LEO TOLSTOY

How did
it go?

Q   **Isn't marriage an outdated concept?**

A   *Only a quarter of all American families incorporate the traditional family unit of marriage and children, although surveys on couples who cohabit reveal striking behavioral similarities. The www.unmarried.org website reports that 55 percent of different-sex cohabitors get married within five years of moving in together and 41 percent of unmarried partner households have children living with them. Although Susan Maushart argues that women no longer need marriage—"We don't need it financially, reproductively or socially"—sociologist Frank Furstenberg pointed out in* Newsweek *that "Paradoxically, more people today value marriage. They take it seriously. That's why they're more likely to cohabit. They want to make sure before they take the ultimate step."*

Q   **How about feminism and sex?**

A   *Although feminist activists hoped to get women sexual freedom in the '70s, many feel that it actually freed up men's sexuality more than ours. Author Sally Cline argues that orgasms are a "form of manipulated emotional labor which women worked at in order to reflect and maintain men's values." However, writer Naomi Wolf suggests that feminism and love are not incompatible, and notes in* Promiscuities *that, "A curious hostility is directed by women against 'feminists who love too much.'" Childcare muddies the waters. In 2005 the* Harvard Business Review *revealed a surprising statistic: of the 1981 class at Stanford University, 57 percent of women graduates have left the workforce. Equality still has a long way to go.*

42

Get close

Sometimes touching, cuddling, and kissing are more important than intercourse. That's great for cats, but here's how to move it from cozy to rosy.

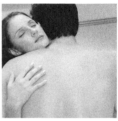

Maybe you're one of those couples that walk everywhere hand in hand and call each other pet names in public. It's obvious your relationship is all about being touchy-feely . . .

If you get too comfortable doing this you could get stuck in the "panda syndrome," a pattern of being affectionate but nonsexual. By nature real pandas are cuddly, but find it hard to mate. Sex therapist Aline P. Zoldbrod explains in her book *Sex Talk*: "For some couples with the Panda Syndrome, kissing, and even genital touching, has become 'nonsexual,' because you have evolved into a pattern where it is understood by each of you that these touches will not progress to sexual excitement. At this point, it is almost impossible for either of you to signal to the other that you want to resume being fully sexual."

This may be a very reassuring position for both of you, especially if you have gained weight or are out of shape: sex is a high-energy activity. Often, though, any apparent sexual passivity is mismatched and one partner may be indulging in masturbation

Here's an idea for you... **To avoid the panda syndrome, develop a code word or phrase, something you wouldn't normally say—like "red fizz"— and use this to indicate that you're feeling positively amorous. You could also experiment with a certain type of kiss that signals the same thing; slipping your tongue in his mouth in a smooch lets him know you want it to go further than a cuddle.**

or finding some other way to get his or her kicks. If you both agree that it's time to get back in the driver's seat for sex, you need to find some way of jerking yourself back into action.

Setting aside an afternoon or evening for pleasure is a good start. If you don't feel like sex yet, then mutual masturbation or oral sex is a sexual activity that's just a zone up from the comfort barrier of cuddling. If even this is too much, at least make your kissing more strident; if you've been doing soft, mushy kisses turn these into passionate ones with tongues.

If you find that touching each other no longer prompts lustful thoughts, it could be that you need some external stimulus. Probably one of the worst things that can happen is for him to buy you some sexy underwear that doesn't fit and that you don't like; it's easier if the woman initiates a sexual interest. Fondle him suggestively when he's in the shower or make your cuddles go a little more in the direction of the genitals. Better still, try to go out more and arouse his interest in a place where you can't easily cuddle and fall into the panda syndrome. For example, go out to dinner and whisper sweet nothings in his ear in the restaurant or pass him suggestive notes. Hopefully, it'll make him anticipate something exciting happening later.

You could also get out of the house more; it's funny how the best way to appreciate your home space is often when you have less of it. Go to the movies, theater, dance, or musicals. You're bound to encounter semi-naked, good-looking people in a state of undress. Another neutral way to initiate an interest is to go to a large bookstore where you can sit and browse the books together. The selection that you pick out should be more daring than normal to encourage your partner to take more of an interest. Have a look at sex manuals or erotic photo books. Sex shops are also great for arousing curiosity—suddenly you've just got to try out that strawberry and champagne lick-off body sauce.

The advantage of going out is that inevitably you buy or find something that piques your interest, which can set a chain of thought going on the way home. Suddenly you are no longer settling for a comfortable night in, but knowing conspirators ready to let loose the moment the door is closed and the curtains are drawn. Enjoy your new sexual adventures!

A good way for cuddling couples to become more sexual is to use their comfortableness together as a prelude to foreplay. See IDEA 5, _Slippery when wet._

Try another idea...

"When things don't work well in the bedroom, they don't work well in the living room either."
DR. WILLIAM MASTERS, sex researcher

Defining idea...

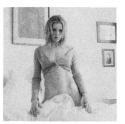

How did
it go?

Q   **Even the idea of sex seems absurd. Is it just an age thing?**

A   *No. Women's sexual desire increases with age, does not peak until the mid-thirties, and continues into menopause and beyond. A survey by the National Council on Aging and the American Association for Retired Persons showed that of 1,000 men and women over fifty, 60 percent were satisfied with their sex lives. An amazing 61 percent said that sex was as good as or better than when they were young! Try doing a bit more exercise to get your blood circulation moving and work on your fantasy life. A good way to tease your partner is to send them a customized fantasy through www.pillowmail.com.*

Q   **After having a baby my body is no longer receptive to sexual feelings. Is this normal?**

A   *Yes, according to several Nerve.com columnists who dared to speak out. In Prude Awakening Lisa Carver writes about how she totally changed after birth. "For a decade and a half, sex had been the main component of my career, even of my personality. Then it was gone without a trace. Doing it seemed as compelling an idea as, say, jumping up and down fourteen times mid-dinner: there was nothing wrong with it, but it just didn't seem to make any sense." When you breastfeed it releases oxytocin, the same chemical that you get from an orgasm, so you feel less sexual.*

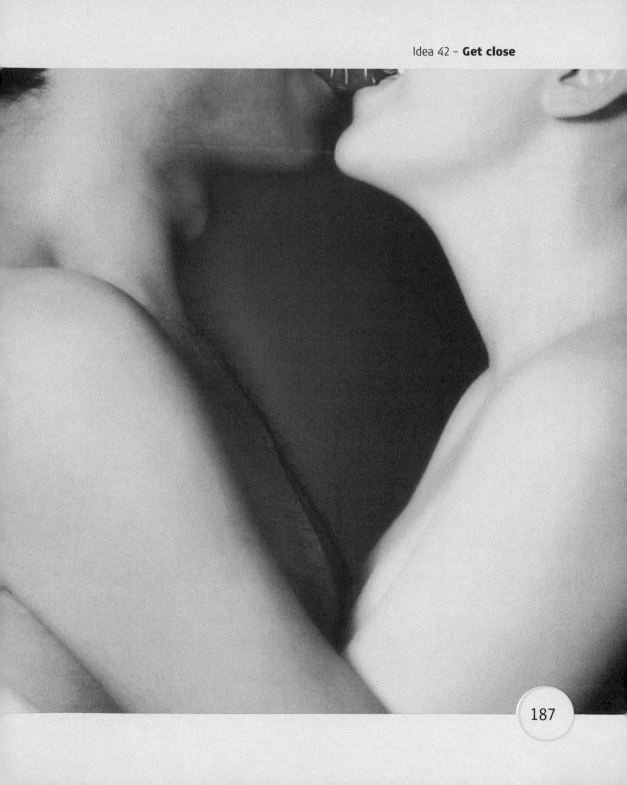

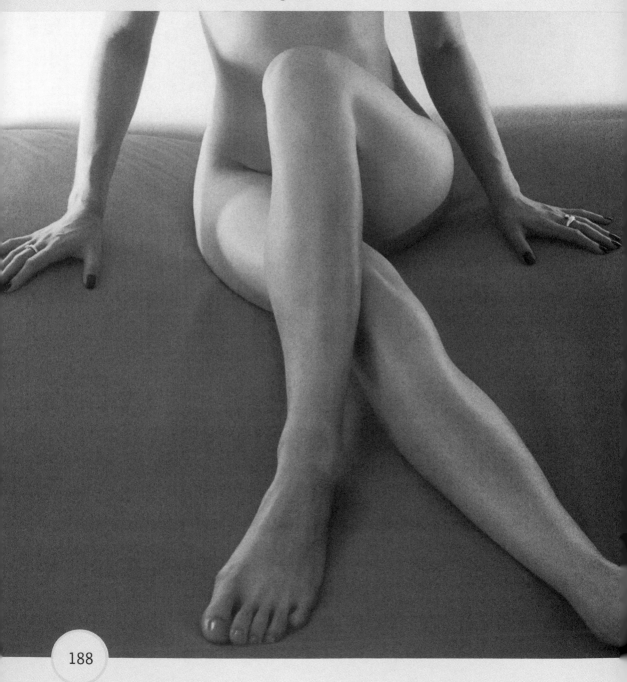

43

First time

You don't have to have sex to be fulfilled. There is a lot of evidence showing that delaying sex until you are ready for it makes for more satisfying orgasms.

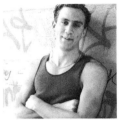

Virginity is becoming fashionable again. It's OK to delay sex, or not to have sex, but your first experience can affect your sexual development, so look before you leap.

Studies show that we're having sex younger, but it's not necessarily better sex. The Kinsey Institute recently revealed that the average age for an American woman to lose her virginity is sixteen, but the average age she experiences her first orgasm is just over twenty! The National Survey of Sexual Attitudes and Lifestyles 2000 showed that many people regret teenage sexual activity; four in five women who had sex at thirteen or fourteen wished they had waited until they were older. In another study, even a third of boys regretted losing their virginity too early. Many girls who become teenage mothers as a result of underage sex have never even had an orgasm.

The first time you have sex is one of the biggest influences on your sexual future, so if you're going to do it make sure that it's a good experience. In a Handbag.com

Here's an idea for you...

Try masturbating at the same time for three consecutive days. How long does it take to get to a state where you can't stop? If you're considering sex with a partner, you'll be able to compare your arousal state, and until you reach that point don't go any further—you're unlikely to orgasm if you do.

article Tracey Cox says, "If losing your virginity was a positive experience, you're more likely to view sex as something that's healthy and enjoyable; the reverse if the experience was a nightmare." Studies show that women who have underage sex have fewer orgasms in later life than women who lose their virginity later, at sixteen to eighteen. It's a difficult time for today's teens. We're saturated with media images of sex and contraception opportunities, so often we end up pressured into having sex too soon. Our changing bodies don't help things either. In *The Sexual Century* Tom Hickman explains, "Two hundred years ago, the mean average onset of puberty was seventeen; today it is eleven years and four months."

Defining idea...

"Writing a book is like having sex for the first time. You should have taken your time and enjoyed it more."
IRVINE WELSH

Naomi Wolf wrote about growing up as a teenager in the '70s in hedonistic San Francisco in *Promiscuities: A Secret History of Female Desire.* She found herself trapped in a virgin/whore dichotomy, which translated simply as "Virgin? What's your problem? Whore? What's your number?" What she and her friends were missing was some kind of ritual or rite of passage that acknowledged they had entered the state of being a nubile young woman: "Other cultures have had the wisdom we have lost about the psychic need to incorporate girls into womanhood through ritual and public transformation." In the West, we're left to cope by ourselves and many of us are simply confused about our sexual desires and what to do about them.

With rising statistics for teenage pregnancies, HIV, and STDs, it's not surprising that some are making celibacy and virginity personal choices. Organizations like True Love Waits encourage people to pledge to abstain from sex until marriage. Others just wait for the right time. Sarah Hinlicky writes in *Subversive Virginity* about how opting out leaves her free from sexual power games: "It escapes the ruthless cycle of winning and losing because it refuses to play the game."

If you've lost your virginity, be sure to read IDEA 32, *Your sexual profile*, to find out if your sexual history reveals anything about your sexual "blueprint."

Try another idea...

Of course, being a virgin doesn't mean you don't get to have orgasms. On the contrary, you're more likely to masturbate and perfect the art of doing this. If you're able to do this yourself, you're much more likely to have a better sexual frisson with someone else. Debra Boxer wrote an extremely erotic Nerve.com essay, "Innocence in Extremis," about being a virgin at the age of twenty-eight. Here she describes a particularly satisfying masturbation experience: "After, my hands shake as if I'd had an infusion of caffeine. I press my hand, palm down, in the vale between my breasts, and it feels as if my heart will burst through my hand."

Do whatever is right for you, but don't engage in sex if you don't get to orgasm. Finally, do indulge in masturbation—it's the ultimate safe sex experience.

"Youth and (until recently) virginity have always been 'beautiful' in women since they stand for experiential and sexual ignorance."
NAOMI WOLF

Defining idea...

How did it go?

Q   Isn't it uncool to be a virgin these days?

A   *Opinions differ, but it seems perverse if there are teenage mothers who have never even had an orgasm. Aldous Huxley called chastity "the most unnatural of all the sexual perversions." Voltaire said, "It is an infantile superstition of the human spirit that virginity would be thought a virtue and not the barrier that separates ignorance from knowledge." The writer P. D. James said, somewhat cynically, "If our sex life were determined by our first youthful experiments, most of the world would be doomed to celibacy. In no area of human experience are human beings more convinced that something better can be had if only they persevere." Virginity is a choice that isn't necessarily passive.*

Q   Any tips on good ways to lose your virginity?

A   *It's better if you've been able to masturbate yourself to orgasm first, and have had some kind of prior passionate relationship with the person involved. Most couples progress from kissing to petting and so on in the weeks leading up to losing your virginity. Get what you can out of frottage (rubbing against each other while fully clothed) before you take your clothes off. Choose a safe place and spend the day with your lover beforehand. Use plenty of lubricant and practice safe sex. Go slow and try to make the moment last: it's a special occasion!*

44

The rake

You know he's bad for you, but you can't resist the impulse . . . Why we've got the hots for the bad ones.

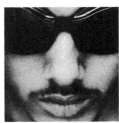

Deep down it's the thrill of no holds barred, testosterone-fueled sex that attracts us to devil-may-care types. They're assertive, exciting, and glamorous—do you want a piece of the action?

Psychologists tell us we're attracted to these aggressive, renegade alpha males because back in the Stone Age we needed prime hunter-gatherer material to bring home the bacon. This may be true, but these days the lure of wild passion is also a significant factor, especially if it's in a relationship that will be long enough to experiment sexually, but not *too* long—we don't want complacency to set in. Before I finally dated the archetypal "bad boy," I'd carefully picked long-term partners for years and years. It was a relief to finally let go and date the type of guy I'd studiously avoided; the doomed "it can't last" element to it only made each moment more exciting.

Here's an idea for you...

Write down the actual benefits your own bad guy has brought to your sex life. You might be surprised at how little you've experimented so far, so why not come up with your own list? After all, you might as well take full advantage of what's available.

Check your real motivations though; many women hope to "reform" bad guys, but in reality they want to break the mold of their own contrite existence. The psychologist Dr. Stovall says, "A 'good girl' is a woman who has followed the rules all of her life; she's been taught to go along with the status quo of what everyone else thinks she should do, be, and want. These women have not had an opportunity to be who they are, so they are attracted to the men who rebel against the rules, and they live vicariously through them." Perhaps what you really need is better, hotter sex but you're afraid of initiating this yourself. After all, we're attracted to people who share similar characteristics with us, so isn't this really you exploring your own wild side?

If your longing for a bad guy is just a cover for your pent-up desires, it's better for you to play this out yourself rather than waiting passively for someone to do it for you. (Bad boys are notorious, a bit like married men, for promising the world then failing to deliver.) Start by sending out the kind of signals that reflect your real personality. If you want to wear that short skirt, even though it doesn't look "respectable," just do it. Even if you need to wear something conservative to work, you can wear naughty undies underneath. Some people have a provocative tattoo to ensure that the part of themselves it represents can never go undercover.

Defining idea...

"The good boys I met typically had the depth of an ashtray. I wanted a misguided angel, a leader of the pack."
ELLEN MILLER, novelist

Remember you need to unlock your own feelings, with the bad guy as an aide, rather than a bind.

Perhaps what you're really hankering after is to become a "bad girl" in your own right. Try being a little predatory: check out IDEA 48, *Sex as sport*.

Try another idea...

Pay attention to your fantasy life. What really turns you on? And what's stopping you from carrying it out? Don't forget he's the mirror to what you want, not the key to the mysteries of the universe. If you make the focus on you, and why you're attracted to him, it'll allow you to lick all the cream without getting sucked in. Don't fall in love—well, not too deeply anyway—as bad boys are emotionally immature and will hurt you if you want them too much. They should be regarded as playthings for a rainy day, and accepted as the risk they are. Enjoy the insights they bring you, but remember they're bound to let you down eventually.

Of course, some of us enjoy the bittersweet finale. Feminist critic Naomi Wolf is surprisingly indulgent about them in *Promiscuities*: "In art as in literature, in film and on the mass-culture page, those desirable bad boys are always in the act of riding away, leaving behind the indulgent feminine consensus on their rottenness and their appeal. The 'victims' recover slowly, tending their wounds, but the irresistible nature of the bad boys' glamour means that those women receive a sympathy not unmixed with envy." Yep, we love 'em, but we don't need them; they're a prop to help us find our own wild side.

"There is always some madness in love. But there is also always some reason in madness."
FRIEDRICH NIETZSCHE

Defining idea...

How did
it go?

Q   Why should I bother with someone like this?

A   *You don't have to. In fact, many women are turning their back on this type.
In* A Modern Girl's Guide to Dynamic Dating *Sarah Ivens says, "Modern
women are too busy to pursue the stereotypical bastard. In between forging
ahead in our careers, keeping up with friends, and staying healthy and
gorgeous, we don't have time to chase after pointless men." However, some
women are inevitably attracted to the wrong type. Some seek the freedom
such a rebel offers; others have had a negative father figure who made
them feel inadequate. They've normalized this behavior and seek it out.
Other women just relish the challenge!*

**Q   Aren't men like this potentially dangerous for our emotional well-
being?**

A   *Yes and no. Of course, most "bad boys" are just insecure guys hiding under
a mask. A small minority, however, are real sociopaths and their inability to
emotionally relate could be deadly. In Brett Easton Ellis's* American Psycho
*Patrick Bateman is suave but nonetheless a serial killer. It's his emotional
blankness that allows him to do such things. "To Evelyn our relationship
is yellow and blue, but to me it's a gray place, most of it blacked out,
bombed . . ." But on the other hand, he represents an extreme case and it's
the scent of danger that can make someone extra attractive. Really you
have to weigh the benefits you're getting against the risk, but assess this
based on your own self-discovery, not his.*

45

Asian secrets

Sex as culture. Steep yourself in the mysterious wonders of the Far East, where not coming is the goal.

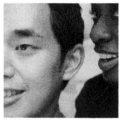

Being able to breathe deeply and exhale this breath from deep inside helps you to focus your energy, connect with your partner, and relax into an amazing, pure energy orgasm.

Tantric sex can be traced back 6,000 years to Ancient China in the form of Taoism. As early as 500 BC the Chinese Tao/Dao studied "injaculation" where men divert their orgasm into their spine and in doing so supposedly retain their energy. One of its advantages was that equal attention was paid to female orgasm, although the men's motives were not selfless, as it was believed that male sexual energy (yang) was precious and needed to be saved. Women's yin was infinite and had the power of immortality. That's why there's so much emphasis on female ejaculation and a penis lingering (even when soft) in the vagina. Although the Chinese were the first to initiate Tantric practices as well as the first sex manuals, the Hindu revival and addition of a spiritual dimension has remained the most popular form, and lots of couples are now getting into Tantric sex and yoga.

Here's an idea for you... **Take a leaf out of the *Kama Sutra* and get him to massage your feet during intercourse. Lie on your back and get your partner to enter you with his knees open around your thighs. In the Pressed Position you lift your butt onto his lower legs and he caresses your feet as he enters you. In the Half Pressed Position, one leg is stretched straight out so you can stimulate your clitoris, too, all at the same time.**

Although you can practice the meditation and breathing rituals at home in readiness for Tantric sex, it's best to combine this with a yoga, meditation, or spiritual class to help prepare your mind. Sexuality is only meant to be one component of the Tantra, not its raison d'être.

Beginning couples can start by bathing together to relax each other, looking deeply into each other's eyes, and performing loving rituals like shampooing hair or cleansing. To maintain your energy levels, arrange healthy snacks on small plates to nibble on as you relax together. For the next stage, move to a sensuous environment, such as cushions on the living room floor, or a bedroom that has been prearranged with candles, incense sticks, or flowers to help you relax. Next, use essential oils like sandalwood or bergamot and take turns gently massaging each other. If you like, you can experiment with touch and gently tease your partner with feathers, velvet, silk, or any texture that feels good on the skin. Don't place too much emphasis on the genitals yet; play with every area of the skin. The aim is to feel relaxed and open to a meditative state.

Now you need to practice your breathing to begin the meditation. If you are supple, try sitting in an open lotus position facing each other, or just sit comfortably using cushions to get your heads at about the same height. The aim is to activate your energy centers. These are known as chakras and the six main ones are at the base of the spine, near the navel, heart, throat, the "third eye" (between the eyes), and the genitals. Try to breathe, concentrate on your genitals and expel your breath out in the direction of your vagina. Both of you should be concentrating on doing this, and when you feel it's working look at each other and try to change the flow of the energy. Take the imaginary breath from your genitals and imagine breathing it into your partner's heart.

Having strong PC muscles is essential to be able to control your orgasmic reflexes. See IDEA 18, *Sexercise.*

Try another idea...

You can use visualization techniques, breathing, and focus to attain a state of deep relaxation, and then in this state you can begin foreplay and sex. You're aiming to make sexual contact much more than genital stimulation, so try to feel as if you are making love to the whole of your partner's body.

To prolong lovemaking and withhold ejaculation, just before the point of no return flex your PC muscles tight and hold the position. The feeling of needing to orgasm should subside slightly, and then you can resume. Both you and your partner can try this advanced trick. The real deal, though, is the meditation side: focus that breath!

"He who realizes the truth of the body can come to know the truth of the universe."
RATNASARA, prophet

Defining idea...

199

How did
it go?

Q   I just want to have great sex! What's the point in meditating?

A   *It's good that you're so enthusiastic, but there's a philosophy and culture that precedes this practice and meditation is the key to getting there. You're actually aiming to let go of ego-driven genital sex and embrace the whole body. Suzie Heumann says on tantra.com, "Most Westerners will only investigate the sexual aspects of Tantra, though the richer areas involve great personal evolution through consciousness. The sexual aspects give us practices that teach us focus and consciousness using sexuality as the vehicle." Some view the recent Western adoption of Buddhist techniques for better sex more cynically; writers like Tessa Bartholomeusz argue that the current vogue for "neo-orientalism" is just a way of getting instant gratification. Either way, even amateurs attempting Tantra will indulge in extended foreplay—never a bad thing!*

Q   Was the Ancient Tantra tradition female positive, then?

A   *Perhaps more so than other cultures, but parts of it were not female friendly. Homosexual activity was considered sacred, but not the union between two women. Jonathan Margolis says in* O: The Intimate History of the Orgasm, *"Married women who indulged in lesbianism, however, were not tolerated by the early Tantric cultists. They were supposed to be punished by being shaved bald, having the two relevant fingers cut off and being led through the town on an ass."*

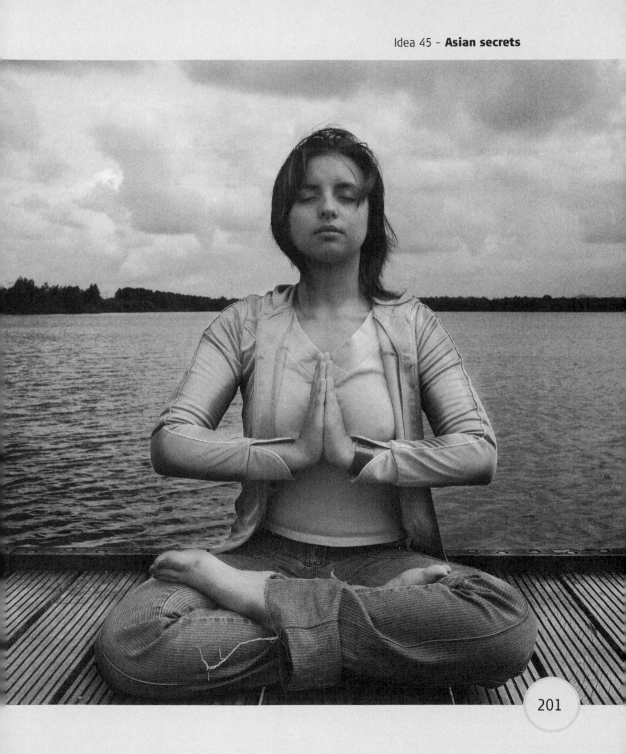

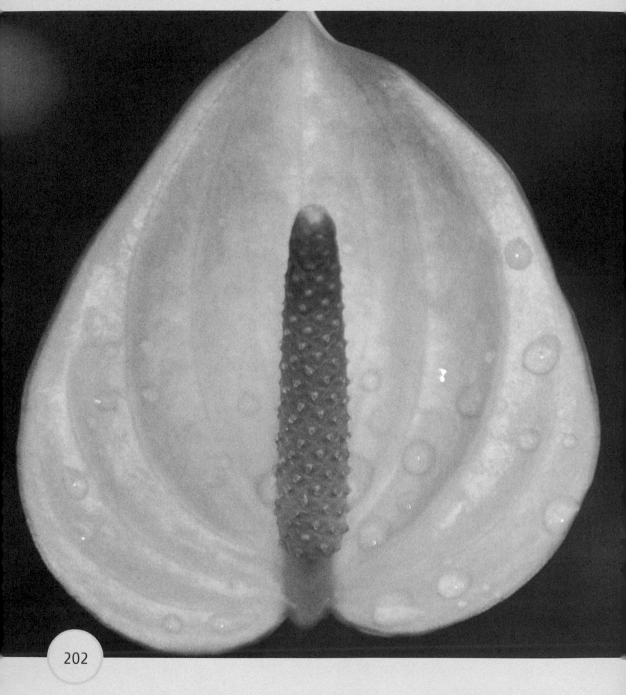

46

Fertility rites

Getting hot about conception and why people do all those weird things on May 1st.

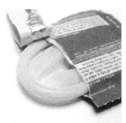

In modern life, we've separated the idea of sex as pleasure from baby making. This is a shame, as the fertility rites from our ancestors were fun and celebrated women.

You've probably spent so long *avoiding* pregnancy that it comes as a bit of a culture shock when you try to conceive. Part of the problem is that our "civilized" culture doesn't really value or ritualize this essential process. Our fertility is taken for granted, something we rarely associate with being a woman, yet for centuries our ability to procreate was essentially what made us sexy. Part of the fun here is trying to recapture the sense of ritual and mystery, and to put a bit of the animal in all of us into our ardor.

Animals know when the female is "hot," but humans have lost this instinct. The knowing woman is aware that when her cervical mucus (creamy stuff seen on underwear/toilet paper) becomes clear, like egg white, then she is ovulating. Women who are more fertile simply have a longer phase of this fertile-quality cervical fluid;

Here's an idea for you...

Around the time you ovulate, get some pink and white flowers to adorn your boudoir to focus your mind on fertility. Get a new translucent slip to get into that goddess feeling; think yourself positively sensual.

in our twenties we have about five days, but this trickles down to just one or two days in our thirties. The good news is that in modern Western society women have more periods and therefore more chances to get a bun in the oven. Endocrinologist Dr. Bruce Carr reckons we have about 450 periods in our lifetime, compared to a mere 50 for women in the Stone Age.

Finding the right moment to time sex for conception is not so difficult. Chart your waking temperature to see when you typically ovulate (your temperature rises after ovulation), or use an ovulation kit that detects the magnificent surge of luteinizing hormone that literally thrusts your egg out of the ovary. The problem is, with only a 10–15 percent chance of getting pregnant per cycle, you run the risk of performing on demand getting a little tedious for both of you.

You could try incorporating some of the old pagan fertility rites into your lovemaking. Our ancestors ritualized the process and repeated it at regular intervals. For example, May Day (also known as Beltane or Walpurgis Night) celebrates the flowering of new life in an explicitly sexual way. The Maypole is a phallic symbol and its ribbons represent the goddess (or maybe multiple female partners) that need to come together in the dance. Other pagan fertility rites include

Defining idea...

"We are no longer—if we ever really were—goddesses or priestesses or queens of our own sexuality. But we want to be."
NAOMI WOLF

washing your face in the dew on the night of April 30 (or even rolling in it naked!), getting your hair wet in rain, having sex outdoors (OK, this is illegal now, but you've got a tent, haven't you?). You can also make a wish as you jump over a bonfire or candle flame for luck. In Germany, communities "dance in the May" and there's even a centuries-long tradition of the "witches' dance" on a remote mountain called the Brocken. Feel free to use any of these practices as your own kinky ritual around the days when you ovulate. At the very least you could watch the cult film *The Wicker Man*, which features some pretty savage fertility rites, but also celebrates nubile and pregnant women in a series of lingering shots.

For info on monitoring your signs of fertility, check out IDEA 3, *Sticky fingers*.

Try another idea...

You can really do anything that makes both the occasion and you feel special. Some people brew their own fertility potions (red clover is said to be good), wear fertility jewelery with particular runes, or make fertility oil. (A potent penis rub is 2 oz of vegetable oil with the contents of one vitamin E capsule, 3 drops of allspice, 3 drops of ylang ylang, and 5 drops of vanilla.) Remember, originally we made blood sacrifices to female deities, and even though you don't need to go quite that far, it's worth making a bit of an effort.

"Take the flame inside you
Burn and burn below
Fire seed and fire feed
And make the baby grow."
THE WICKER MAN

Defining idea...

How did
it go?

Q   Surely these rituals are outdated?

A   Feminist writer Naomi Wolf argues that "girls need better rites of passage in our culture" because the compartmentalization of sex versus conception is damaging for us. Way back in 1948 anthropologist Margaret Mead found that different cultures make alternative sexual experience seem normal. Stephen Beckerman found that up to the middle of the last century the Canela women in Amazonian Brazil had sex with multiple partners when they wanted a baby and believed every man's sperm added a bit to the mix. It's interesting that in preliterate cultures today, where the connection between sex and conception is not understood, women have more power. It's when men grasp their paternity rites that the problems start.

Q   Is female orgasm important for conception?

A   Yes. In Sperm Wars *Robin Baker suggests that "to maximize conception, a woman should experience an orgasm immediately after a man ejaculates." Psychologist David Buss from the University of Texas says in* The Evolution of Desire, *"Women on average eject roughly 35 percent of the sperm within thirty minutes of the time of insemination. If the woman has an orgasm, however, she retains 70 percent of the sperm and ejects only 30 percent." Orgasm also conveniently produces the chemical oxytocin, which encourages us to lie still and helps things along, but it will only work if fertile-quality cervical fluid is present.*

47

Hedonism

Do you have a wild streak? Make sure that you really have fun if you play hard. Here's a cautionary exposé of the real sex lives of the Hollywood goddesses.

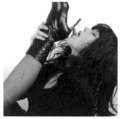

Don't believe all the hype. Most of the women promoted as sex goddesses actually had dysfunctional sex lives and didn't always reach the magic O.

Many of the Hollywood goddesses were international sex symbols but did not use their famed desirability to have the most wonderful sexual experiences (despite what their publicists would have us believe). Indeed, many of them never or rarely climaxed: Jean Harlow said the physical act made her sick; sex was an "inescapable burden that women had to endure" for Marlene Dietrich; Marilyn Monroe rarely, if ever, had an orgasm; and Lana Turner admitted in her autobiography *Lana: The Lady the Legend, the Truth*, "I might as well confess that I was not a great companion in bed . . . Sex was so much what I symbolized, so much of my image, that I closed myself off to the pleasures of the act." Positive proof that the way that you look is not the same as the way you feel.

Here's an idea for you... **Imagine you are a famous movie star, and tell your partner that you want to act out her role. Tell him imperiously to meet you at a certain time and/or location and dress appropriately. As the sexiest woman in the world, dream up a list of things you'd like to do to the next man who courts your favor. Borrow trademark sexual habits or style tips and have a ball!**

If you want to have a good sex life, avoid making the mistakes that the Hollywood goddesses did. It's no surprise that they had unusual lifestyles; people who are motivated to become famous are often suffering from complexes that they perceive their public recognition will compensate for. Many female stars are sexually outrageous because, for women, antisocial behavior is often expressed in sexually provocative behavior, whereas men become aggressive.

The legendary stars were typically into exhibitionism and even notoriously shy Greta Garbo liked to garden in the nude. Hedonist Tallulah Bankhead took her clothes off at every opportunity and often met people for the first time while on the toilet or sitting in the bathtub. Monroe said, "I am only comfortable when I am naked" and referred to her body as "my magic friend." If you're into exhibitionism, ask yourself what motivates you to get naked. If it's for shock value, you're probably not getting the optimum sexual benefit out of it.

Defining idea... *"I can never say no."*
TALLULAH BANKHEAD

Another star tendency is to have indiscriminate sex with both men and women (Bankhead boasted she had over 5,000 partners). Louise Brooks was fired at the age of fifteen from her job in a dance troupe because she had slept with all of the backstage crew.

Joan Crawford had worked as a stripper and prostitute and tried to seduce fellow actresses by getting them to try on her dresses and making a move on them if they undressed.

For a closer look at insecurity and fame see IDEA 4, *The beautiful and the bad.*

Try another idea...

Both Marilyn Monroe and Jean Harlow tried to overcome their sexual frustrations at not being able to come by a series of anonymous sex sprees where they would pick up men and hope they would not be recognized. According to Nigel Cawthorne in *Sex Lives of the Hollywood Goddesses*, Marilyn Monroe "told her maid that she would go with anyone, irrespective of their looks, provided they were 'nice.'" Similarly, at a low point in her career, "Jean [Harlow] took to drinking and she would forget who she slept with, what they did with her, and where they went in the morning . . . Often she would not bother to remove her clothes, so that she could get on to the next one quicker in the frantic hope that she would become pregnant." If you have a hectic love life, make sure that you actually enjoy your amorous encounters.

It's sad, but many of the stars who were into hedonistic behavior paid a high price for their fun. They had multiple abortions. Tallulah Bankhead had to have a hysterectomy at the age of thirty-one due to gonorrhoea; Clara Bow drifted in and out of mental institutions and died a recluse; and many developed problems due to alcohol and drug addictions. It just goes to show that being a sex symbol doesn't qualify you for good sex; in fact, quite the opposite.

Defining idea...

"I will always believe that youth and beauty are, to a great extent, fuel to be burned in pursuit of pleasure rather than fruit to be preserved at all costs for a rainy day."
JULIE BURCHILL

How did it go?

Q   What has all this got to do with my sex life?

A   *Surveys show that 90 percent of women feel worse about their own self-image after flicking through a women's magazine where they are confronted by perfect-looking, airbrushed models. Similarly, the images of Hollywood goddesses can make us feel inadequate because we don't look, move, or talk like them. Therapist Aline P. Zoldbrod says in* Sex Talk, *"Lots of people, women especially, are operating under the misconception that their lover is turned on or off based on how she looks. The truth of the matter is, studies find it is how a lover 'responds' sexually, not how he or she looks, that makes them sexually attractive and memorable to their lover." So concentrate on feeling sexy, rather than looking the part.*

Q   Are you saying that being hedonistic is a bad thing?

A   *No, but if we're having sex supposedly for pleasure, it doesn't make sense to do what Monroe and Harlow did and pick up partners just for the hell of it, encounters which presumably didn't even result in a climax. There are legendary hedonists, like the real Cleopatra, who appeared to have reveled in their pursuit of pleasure (although her downfall was her fondness for Roman generals). Whatever you do, do it for your benefit, and ensure that your personal safety and sexual health are not unduly compromised.*

48

Sex as sport

Doing a tour of one-night stands? Making the most of flexible friends after dark.

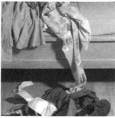

These days casual sex is an exciting alternative to traditional relationships. It can be an emotional minefield though, so here's how to have the spark without getting burned.

The route toward full sexual intercourse is getting quicker. It's common for people to fall into bed on the first date, regardless of whether the affair ends up as a one-off or a full-blown relationship. However, if you don't communicate, you won't know what you're getting into. You could end up hurt if what you thought was the start of a new relationship fizzles out, or annoyed if a conquest keeps phoning for dates and you don't want that, so establish what you want at the outset. Judging by how many women are logging on to Craigslist.com with its notorious Casual Encounters section for "one-off, no ties, no-nonsense sex," there are a lot of women out there who just want that and we're becoming increasingly better at getting it.

One of the bonuses about deciding to go ahead with the chase for casual sex is that you don't know when it's going to happen. That means lots of anticipatory

Here's an idea for you... **If you don't want to go all the way, restrict yourself to kissing someone passionately in a public street. You avoid the risk of bringing someone home or going to their place, and it gives you a dry run to see how you feel about casual dating.**

pleasure, soaking in luxurious baths, attending to matters of depilation, and wearing knock 'em dead underwear. Just thinking about the possibility gives you a boost and any extra effort you've made will increase your confidence. It's better to find someone who is not particularly connected to you or your friends (not a work colleague, your friend's ex, a neighbor). At the same time, picking up a complete stranger comes with its own risks (he could be a psychopath) and you risk him knowing where you live if he goes back to your place.

Good meeting places for casual sex are nightclubs, bars, and concerts, but really any social gathering offers opportunities if you're not too shy to look for them. The advantage of seeking out a casual partner is that you can discount a lot of the attributes you'd look for in a long-term partner, and can go for attractiveness and sex appeal over a good sense of humor. There's also not very much to lose, so you're not ruining anything by flirting actively. If he's not interested you'll get the message. As long as you tell someone where you're going (should anything occur) and have got your little bag of tricks handy (containing essentials like condoms, clean underwear, makeup, cell phone) you're free to take advantage of what's offered.

It's a good idea to kiss him intensely first before making up your mind. You can tell a lot about a man from the way he kisses. Dance with him if possible: does his body respond well to yours? Also bring up the subject of safe sex before you've dragged him away anywhere. Get the basics out of the way: where you're going, contraception, if you're sleeping over.

Flirting is an art in itself and is a gentle, playful way to feel sexy. Being able to do it well is a great way to pick someone up, so check out IDEA 24, Dangerous liaisons.

Try another idea...

Many one-night stands are fueled by alcohol, which is a big passion killer, so don't get too wasted. Ideally, once you're in a suitable location, you should be able to pick up where you left off. Initiate things by kissing and hugging first. Aim to give and receive as much foreplay as possible (lousy conquests lead to rushed orgasms, and their benefits are largely psychological). Talk dirty if it turns you on, and don't be afraid to use any sex toys you have with you, or to experiment with anal sex or different positions. In *Brief Encounters*, Emily Dubberley says, "Just because you're having casual sex, it doesn't mean that you have to keep things vanilla."

Don't turn cold as soon as you've come, but don't expect roses either. Discretion is everything. If you've made it clear there's no commitment, don't be afraid to be affectionate or enjoy multiple orgasms. It's meant to be fun!

"One should be a sex maniac, but one should never be indiscriminate."
CYNTHIA HEIMEL, author

Defining idea...

How did
it go?

Q   Isn't having one-night stands destructive for my self-esteem?

A   *On the one hand, it's good to feel you can do it if you want to. In* Friends
and Enemies, *Dorothy Rowe says, "Being seen to be sexually active is now a
measure of success." Many women are paying for sex escorts, and enjoying
longer-term relationships with "friends with benefits." On the other hand,
Emily Dubberley says in her book* Brief Encounters, *"One-night stands are
also the easiest way to get a bad reputation." It's a numbers game: maybe
a handful is OK, but anything over twenty seems greedy. Avoid getting into
a repetitive cycle of doing it if it doesn't make you feel good. Lucy Grealy
suffered from low esteem because of facial cancer that left her face scarred.
In her* Autobiography of a Face, *she reveals, "Bent on proving I was
desirable, I started collecting lovers, having a series of short-term
relationships that always ended, I was certain, because I wasn't beautiful
enough. I became convinced that anyone who wanted to have a real
relationship with me was automatically someone I didn't want." Don't get
into this!*

Q   Do women have more fun in one-night stands?

A   *Difficult one. You can't get too kinky; stuff like bondage is too dangerous
with a stranger. When* Redbook *magazine did a 100,000-reader response
survey in 1977 they concluded that women who were more adventurous
and experimental had fewer orgasms than women who were married!*

49

Power to the people

The whip and the flesh, inside the world of S&M. The pleasure of pain and sweet submission.

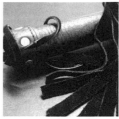

Images of kink are everywhere. Most of the time they are used to shock in advertising, but experimenting along the edges of your "shadow selves" can lead to mind-opening experiences.

Making love doesn't have to be restricted to "vanilla." Every relationship is a power exchange, whether you're conscious of it or not, so it makes sense to play around with the boundaries of it a little. The biggest turnoff couples face engaging in "regular" sex is a lack of communication about initiating new elements into their love play. The good news is that to get into S&M games you have to spend more time discussing your likes and dislikes before doing anything. If nothing else, at least it will get you talking. You also get to experiment with dressing up, different toys, and implements—mind-broadening activities in themselves.

In *Sensuous Magic* Patrick Califia says, "There are a lot of details to be determined—when and where the scene will take place, what roles will be adopted, limits (that

The next time you are in the middle of foreplay, ask your partner to put his hands behind his head and close his eyes while you tickle him with something soft and silky. At any time he can open his eyes or release his hands, so there's no pressure. If this works, you can progress on to more exciting things . . .

is, what specific activities can or should not happen), what safe word to use (a code word that can be used to stop the action), whether or not there will be genital sex, what kind of birth control to use . . ." He suggests writing down three different lists—one for things you definitely like, one for activities that are taboo, plus a list of maybes. Even people who have fantasized for a long time about an activity don't know how they'll actually feel about doing it until it happens. Always agree on everything first and initiate things slowly; it's a bit like foreplay but with more options!

Things to try include tying someone up (bondage), tickling (with hand or feather), stroking, spanking, caning, and whipping. If you want to try being submissive without all the fancy gear, you can try meting out "school" type punishments. Califia says an easy one is making someone stand next to a wall keeping a piece of gum or a coin in place with their nose. Bondage adds an element of fantasy (it's one of the most common ones for both men and women). Be wary about using makeshift household items like silk scarves; they are actually like wire in the wrong hands. Always pad areas that you want to bind first (handcuffs should also be padded). If in doubt, raid the kitchen for cling film and mummify your victim (don't cover the face and don't leave it on for more than an hour, though); you could try a little light spanking over the wrapping.

"Whether we like it or not, pain grabs and holds our attention in a way that pleasure, with its light, frivolous, playful personality, usually does not."
DAVID RAMSDALE, author

216

Adding a little pain to the proceedings is stimulating for some because it releases endorphins—the same feel-good chemicals we get when we exercise. Too much is a turnoff, though, and everyone has a different pain threshold. Always remember to warm up each part of the body first; before moving on to harder strokes, you could start with stroking, move on to tickling, and progress to hand spanking, then possibly using a different implement. Don't forget that faster strokes feel harder simply because the person experiencing it has less time to catch his breath. So take it slowly and experiment.

Even if you don't have any specific fetishes or S&M fantasies, most people will find it interesting to try both "top" and "bottom" roles. Most newbies will try being a bottom first, and in the "scene" bottoms outnumber tops by ten to one! Although it might seem appealing to be dominant, in actual fact they are doing all the work. They are not doing whatever they want to someone, but working to a pre-agreed "script" that should be mutually fulfilling. In addition, who is penetrated is not determined by the role they are playing. The submissive partner may be "made" to use their mouth/penis on the other, and the dominant partner could accept or initiate sexual activity. The whole point is that it's a game where you invent your own rules. Break free from conventional constraints and find out what really turns you on!

If you're not sure who should be the dominant partner in a scene, take a look at the politics of initiation in IDEA 9, Point of entry.

Try another idea...

"Heavier is not necessarily better. The best kind of sex play is the kind that provides the most mutual pleasures for you and your partner(s)."
PATRICK CALIFIA, author

Defining idea...

217

How did it go?

Q **I want to liven up my sex life without going to extremes! Isn't indulging in S&M only for perverts?**

A *Patrick Califia says, "S&M is an umbrella term that includes many, many sexualities." Some people actively enjoy pain, others don't. It could be that your version of S&M is simply sex with interesting costumes, or a blindfold that tantalizingly applies the thrill of sensory deprivation to your "victim." There's no pressure to conform, because here you are making up all the rules anyway. Deciding what you want and don't want is really the point.*

Q **I tried doing some light spanking on my husband's buttocks and he enjoyed it. He encouraged me to go harder and likes being whipped, but I feel out of my depth. How can I learn new skills?**

A *Lots of ways. You can browse your local sex shop or an online catalog like www.heartwoodwhips.com, www.stockroom.com, or www.stormyleather. com. Your aim is to wake up the area of the skin you are working first and find the "map" of its tender points. What kind of stroke or implement is preferred? Don't apply strokes too quickly and vary and overlap the areas you are working on. The three basic whipping strokes are the forehand, backhand, and the figure eight and you can vary these, along with pressure and frequency.*

50

Wet scenes

Want to use a remote control on your pulse rate? Some of the most extraordinary films on the planet for inspiration.

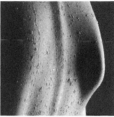

The biggest stumbling block for women is "getting in the mood" in the first place.
A sexy DVD goes a long way into kick-starting something that will inevitably lead to a bit of action.

My grandmother once instructed me to fetch her some library books; they had to be romantic with lots of passion, but nothing *too* sexy! Likewise, we each have our own boundaries. If you think *Last Tango in Paris* is too extreme, don't rent *Anal Bad Girls*. Lots of women use erotica and pornography as straightforward arousal aids, switching them off as soon as the heat of the moment has gone. However, there are films featuring every possible perversion, stuff to tantalize us, as well as films that bring sexual issues to the fore. We can explore film noir, mainstream flicks, and experimental fare, as well as hard-core. Think of them as mind-openers to help you explore new things and open the floodgates to talking about sensitive issues as well as the obvious!

Here's an idea for you...

In mainstream porn it could be that you don't like many of the guys because their main requirement is simply to have a big penis. Try gay porn, where the men will look better (a soft-core example is *Sunshine After the Rain*); it's also a chance to get an insight into a different sexual culture.

Starting gently, some films show nothing but have a powerful erotic charge where unbearable longings surface. Try classic studies of repression like *Black Narcissus* (1947), *Repulsion* (1965), and the Val Lewton–produced famous "B" movies *Cat People* (1942) and *The Seventh Victim* (1943). A stunning film noir is Fuller's *The Naked Kiss* (1964) about a former call girl who goes "straight"; critic Mike LaSalle called it "one of the wisest, slickest and most unorthodox feminist films one could ever hope to see."

If you want to be more upfront, some mainstream films are billed as "erotic" like *Last Tango in Paris* (1972), *Crimes of Passion* (1984), *9½ Weeks* (1986), *Henry and June* (1990), *The Rapture* (1991), *The Pillow Book* (1996), *Boogie Nights* (1997)—and they are stylish to boot. Personally, I'm a sucker for sexy musicals, but not everyone will warm to *Flashdance* (1983), *Showgirls* (1995), or *Coyote Ugly* (2000). There's also art-house erotica that inflames the mind rather than the genitals; try *Belle du Jour* (1968), *The Holy Mountain* (1973), *The Night Porter* (1973), *Immoral Tales* (1974), *In the Realm of the Senses* (1976), *Caligula* (1980), *Blue Velvet* (1986), and *Bitter Moon* (1994). There's also the experimental short, *The Operation* (1995), the first film to be shot entirely in infrared.

Some couples use naughty instructional videos, for example Nina Hartley's various guides, Annie Sprinkle's *Fire in the Valley* (1999), and *Becoming Orgasmic* (1994). Director Andrew Blake's porn films also appeal to couples because his work is stylish, the actors attractive, and the action women-centered: see *Possessions* (1998), *Aria* (2001), and *Hard Edge* (2003). Former porn star Candida Royalle runs Femme, which produces soft porn aimed at women; try *Revelations* (1992), *Eyes of Desire* (1998), and *Stud Hunters: A Hard Man is Good to Find* (2003).

If you're worried about the length of time it takes you to get aroused, check out some tips in IDEA 8, *Starter's orders*.

The original classics that changed the porn industry were *Deep Throat* (1972), *The Devil in Miss Jones* (1972), and *Behind the Green Door* (1972). However, the golden age of porn is 1974–1989 where big budgets and good story lines predominated, as in *The Punishment of Anne* (1975), *Sensations* (1975), *The Opening of Misty Beethoven* (1976), *Pretty Peaches* (1978), *Night Dreams* (1983), *Café Flesh* (1983), *Traci I Love You* (1986), and one of my favorites, *Inside Marilyn* (aka *Inside Olinka*, 1985).

After this period, the industry has been dominated by cheaper video productions, which has allowed for specialized subgenres to develop, such as anal, spanking, bondage, and so on; the Maximum Perversion series is self-explanatory! There's also a growing market for amateur, "homemade" porn. Alongside this, technically advanced directors like Michael Ninn have given us films like *Sex* (1995), *Latex* (1996), and *Garden of Shadows* (2003) that play around with sci-fi and kink using state-of-the-art technology. Some feel this is too clinical, but whatever you're into, there's something to turn you on, so check out your local video store and have a fun night in!

"I want films that install themselves in my sexual imagination by making me feel that sex is a part of life, and at the same time make me feel that sex is an intoxicant, a passage to elsewhere."
JONATHAN LETHEM, novelist

How did it go?

Q   Even though I enjoy watching porn tapes with my boyfriend, I felt betrayed when I found stuff he'd bought alone. Am I being hypocritical?

A   *No. Activist and feminist Tuppy Owens says in* Tales from the Clit, *"I love porn very much. I love looking at it. I work in it. It is my life." But despite her heavy personal involvement, she still felt "a bit of a shock" when a boyfriend furtively used porn (pictures of naked men) to masturbate to. Tuppy is perhaps the most liberal woman on earth, so anyone can feel uncomfortable about coming across something unexpectedly, especially when it represents a fetish/theme you don't share. Tell your partner he can buy anything he wants as long as you know about it.*

Q   Do I really need porn? Why should I need an external stimulus?

A   *If you don't like porn, don't watch it. In this chapter, there are plenty of interesting films that are not hard-core. Don't forget women are often conditioned to feel porn is bad and men are more sexual. This attitude is left over from the Victorians—previously it was women who were considered the rampant ones. Also, it's a bit like the first time you try Stilton cheese or olives. Maybe it's weird at first but you can get used to it, so do see a few movies first before you make up your mind.*

51

Sheer filth

You never realized fun could be this dirty. Maybe you look a little undignified in your quest for passion but, hey, it feels good!

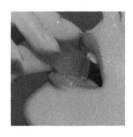

Worrying about how you look, sound, or smell can distract you from having that wonderful orgasm. It really is a case of accepting the rough with the smooth.

Our perception of how we look and taste during sex matters. Some people are put off by insecurities that prevent them from enjoying sex or even having an orgasm at all. In 1999 the Canadian website Queendom.com polled 15,000 adults and found that 46 percent of women who were unable to come blamed a lack of confidence in their appearance. Both men and women can be afraid to let go. In the same survey 61 percent of women and 72 percent of men "lose the plot" when their bodies start grunting and groaning, especially during the final "vinegar strokes." Having good orgasms, then, means lightening up a bit and becoming more body-tolerant.

During sex you have to forget about everything being sterile and prissy clean, even if you've spent hours preparing for the big moment. Sex educator and writer Tuppy

Here's an idea for you... **Practicing "water sports" helps you feel more at ease with your body. Urine is sterile, and if you can let yourself go and actually pee on your partner in the bath or shower (you choose where on his body), you shouldn't have performance anxiety in the throes of orgasm.**

Owens says, "I do love images of people when you see signs of them really being turned on, like bodies which are flushed red, sweating, shaking, dribbling. I like it when people go completely berserk. Shame it's so rare." Real sex is messy; gynecologist Dr. Carol Livoiti points out that our vaginal lips (labia minora) are the sweatiest part of the body and have more sweat glands per inch than our armpits! Dealing with sweat and having to clean up various bodily fluids afterward is part of the game. And for those who enjoy more extreme pleasures, like scarification, fire play, or permanent piercing, there's also damaged skin to tend to afterward. Emily Dubberley, in *Brief Encounters,* says you shouldn't be afraid to open up and tell your partner what you want, even in a situation where it's a one-night stand: "You should also be ballsy enough to take any embarrassing situations in your stride; farts, cramps, and strange odors can all form part of the sex experience, so get used to being blasé about it."

Defining idea... *"We are all in the gutter, but some of us are looking at the stars."*
OSCAR WILDE

Of course, practicing safe sex is the best way to deal with any potential issues. For instance, if you want to finger your partner's anus, using a latex glove makes it easy to clean up afterward without having to scrub your fingernails. Porn actors typically take an enema before any action (although the poo should be out of reach in the colon anyway) and it's reputed that some actors eat very lightly for up to three days before a shoot. We need to become more clued in about safe sex and stop worrying about getting the sheets dirty! For instance, to enjoy anal play, you need a supply of latex gloves and condoms, lots of lubricant, and a trash can in the place where you'll have sex; it doesn't have to be "dirty."

Of course, some people like to be dirty. Napoleon forbade his wife to wash for two weeks before he came home from battle; he loved her natural smell! Men are conditioned by porn to believe women love to be ejaculated on—always stipulate what is acceptable, maybe over your face is fine as long as he avoids your eyes? Some women go to extremes and practice bukkake (they let multiple men masturbate over them). The range of bizarre turn-ons fills a book, *The Encyclopaedia of Unusual Sexual Practices* by Brenda Love. You don't have to do anything extreme, but stop fretting about getting all hot and sweaty.

Being able to deal with all manner of bodily fluids is an essential prerequisite for some of the practices in IDEA 35, *Beyond the beyond*.

Try another idea...

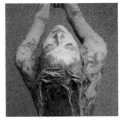

"Today I am dirty, but tomorrow I'll be just dirt."
CARL PANZRAM, serial killer

Defining idea...

How did it go?

Q   I find anything smelly a bit disgusting. What advantage could there be in getting all hot and sticky?

A   *Our sense of smell helps us to pick up on hormonal vibes and can make us more attracted to people! In 2005 researchers at the University of Jyvaskyla in Finland discovered men could sniff out when a woman was ovulating. Forty-two women on the pill and thirty-nine who were not were asked to wear T-shirts for two consecutive nights. Volunteer male "sniffers" were asked to rate which T-shirts smelled best, and the naturally ovulating females (those not on the pill) won hands down—it seems that the men could smell their hormones. Another test in 1986 at the Monell Chemical Senses Center in Philadelphia asked men to wear pads under their armpits to trap their sweat and then froze it and smeared it on the upper lip of female volunteers. Although the women smelled nothing in particular, after fourteen weeks of treatment those with irregular periods had more normal cycles. There is some kind of magic in sweat after all!*

Q   If all this is so natural, why was the missionary position the standard until recently?

A   *Although in the Bible Jesus doesn't speak about sex directly, from AD 342 the Christian church banned sex that did not involve the vagina. Perhaps they wanted us to be fruitful and multiply.*

52

Anticlimax

Dealing with the come down. When you're tingling and glowing, hold that feeling: how to ride the roller coaster of changing emotions.

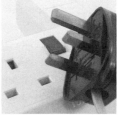

There is some evidence that bareback sex provides extra fringe benefits, but whether you practice safe sex or not, savor the moment and enjoy your anticlimax, too.

The French describe orgasm as *le petit mort* (the little death), which perfectly sums up the feelings of anticlimax and mild disappointment that can come after the first few bursts of pleasure. Mitzi Szereto, editor of an anthology on this theme, says, "Rather than using the term merely as a definition for a pleasurable physiological occurrence, I'm taking *le petit mort* literally, thereby connecting the act of sex with the act of death." Edgy stuff, and that's why it's crucial to kiss and cuddle at the stage of what could be a literal comedown. Of course, having an orgasm brings enormous health benefits and the flow of endorphins helps to relieve anxiety and depression. However, women experience orgasm differently than men. They simply don't have a point of "ejaculatory inevitability" (men will come even if police burst into the room). As Aline P. Zoldbrod explains in *Sex Talk*, "This accounts for why

Here's an idea for you...

After intercourse, avoid instantly rushing off to wipe yourself clean. Instead curl up with your partner and establish a silly ritual that keeps you laughing and cuddling for a good ten minutes. It could be he tells you a "bedtime" story or massages your shoulders. Use something to relax both of you and cherish the moment.

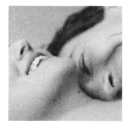

more men than women consider sex to be 'relaxing.'" Very often men feel completely relaxed after sex and want to roll over and fall asleep, whereas women are still reacting to various hormonal and chemical interactions. The sex act for women is not yet over.

Some recent research suggests that sperm can act as an antidepressant and that its contact with the vaginal wall provides a natural high. Dr. Gordon Gallup studied 293 female students at the State University of New York in 2002; those who always had sex without using a condom were quantifiably happier than those who used condoms or didn't have sex. Participants had to answer twenty questions on the Beck Depression Inventory, a standard test used by mental-health professionals. The women who used condoms had the same results as those who were not sexually active, which suggested that it was the actual vaginal/sperm contact that had the effect. In addition, the effects of a sperm "donation" can last up to three days, so it's no wonder that women feel a range of conflicting emotions after contact with what is, in effect, a hormonal douche.

Semen is a very complicated substance—it contains vitamins and follicle-stimulating hormones as well as estrogen and testosterone. Women whose partners come inside them have fewer premenstrual symptoms, and it seems to regulate their ovulation; women who have irregular periods often menstruate like clockwork with regular bareback sex. On the downside, the same women can have withdrawal symptoms if the relationship ends, suggesting a dependency on sperm. Dr. Gallup says in *Semen and Depression*, "It's a chemical dependency—or there's some kind of psychological dependency that's being driven by the presence of semen." Women who use condoms also take longer to form a new sexual relationship.

This does not mean that sperm is the new Prozac or that you should throw caution to the wind, but it does suggest that there is much more at stake when committing to a fluid-bonded relationship. Whatever your status, the way you deal with anticlimax is an important part of love play. Some people come down slowly, still touching and caressing. Tell your

After sex it's a good idea to continue kissing and cuddling; you might even want to go for it again. Learn more about being multiorgasmic in IDEA 16, *Extra credit*.

Try another idea…

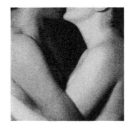

"People who have been much loved retain even in old age a radiating quality difficult to describe but unmistakable. Even a stone that has been blazed on all day will hold heat after nightfall . . ."
DAME ETHYL SMYTH, composer

Defining idea…

229

Defining
idea...

"Some people report a feeling of undefined sadness after orgasm, called post-coital tristesse, which I always thought would make a great name for a rock group."
BARBARA KEESLING, sex therapist and author

partner if it still feels good to have your vagina caressed or not. It could be you have a yearning at this point to have your breasts squeezed. The sex educators Vera and Steve Bodansky recommend putting both palms on the woman's pubic bone and pressing to squeeze the blood out of the genitals and get her to come down more quickly.

Whatever you do, after-love is essential. You can pass tissues to each other, generally fuss over each other, and get him to be the nice one who fetches the cup of tea or turns the light off. Even if you're not remotely romantic, be nice. Coming down can be just as good as going up.

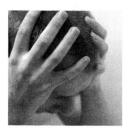
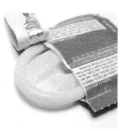

Q **At the moment I'm enjoying casual sex relationships. Is it really appropriate to be "nice" at the end when I'm not planning to see them again?**

How did it go?

A *Yes. It's amazing how straight vanilla heterosexuals manage to bungle the casual sex thing time after time. If you're honest about what you want up front, there should be no awkwardness. You should have already decided if someone's staying or not. Whatever, it's appropriate to give each other a cuddle afterward and maybe share a cup of tea and a cigarette before one of you dashes off. It's also polite to call/text the next day to check that the other person got home safely. If you fall into the habit of being cold directly after you're satiated, you're really only denying yourself part of your rightful pleasure from the experience.*

Q **Are you saying I shouldn't use condoms?**

A *No, that's up to you to decide. There are some benefits to being fluid-bonded, but it's essential for you both to get STD testing done first to establish that this is a practical option. The most important thing is that you both come down from the sexual experience in a supportive way. It could be that you slather each other with ice, snuggle, or have wild oral congress. Just avoid the aircraft landing syndrome—you know, seatbelts off and the inevitable free-for-all struggle to get up and go.*

Where it's at . . .

Index

52 Brilliant Ideas

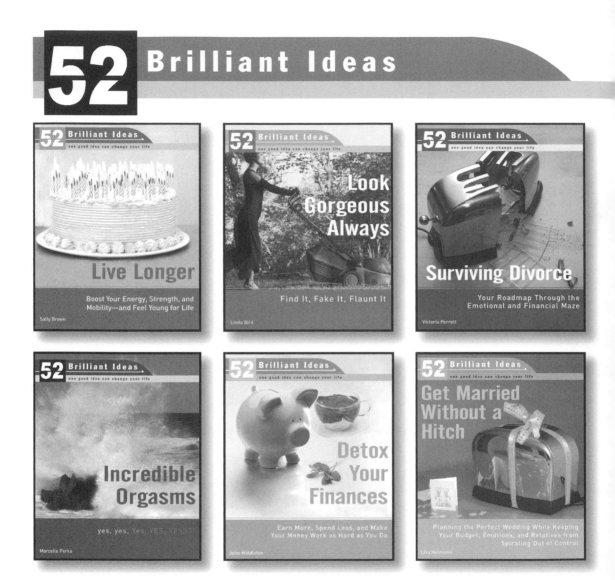

LIVE LONGER
978-0-399-53302-0 • 0-399-53302-8

LOOK GORGEOUS ALWAYS
978-0-399-53304-4 • 0-399-53304-4

SURVIVING DIVORCE
978-0-399-53305-1 • 0-399-53305-2

INCREDIBLE ORGASMS
978-0-399-53303-7 • 0-399-53303-6

DETOX YOUR FINANCES
978-0-399-53301-3 • 0-399-53301-X

**GET MARRIED
WITHOUT A HITCH**
978-0-399-53306-8 • 0-399-53306-0

PERIGEE An imprint of Penguin Group (USA)

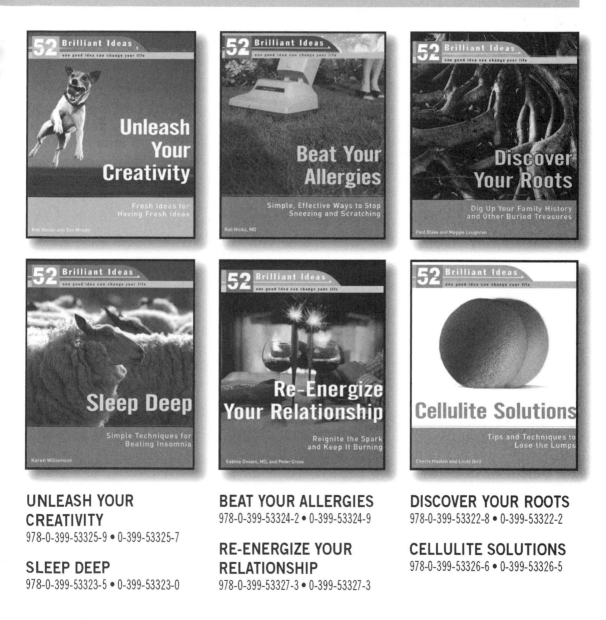

52 fresh ways to ride that wave

From getting aroused more fully to finding "trigger" sexual positions, *Incredible Orgasms* is the perfect guide for any woman who wants to explore her sexuality, body, and libido and get the most out of her sex life.

Filled with advice and ideas to implement tonight, *Incredible Orgasms* covers everything from how to point your lover in the right direction to the latest massage oils, potions, and positions for the most adventurous sexplorers among us.

Idea #10: Classic positions

Idea #13: Toys R no fuss

Idea #14: Alternative erogenous zones

Idea #25: Porn star protocol

Idea #33: Let yourself go

Idea #37: Eyes wide shut

With a mix of the titillating and the time-tested, *Incredible Orgasms* will inspire the romantic and the sexually adventurous alike.

Marcelle Perks is a journalist who has written for a range of publications including the *Guardian*, *British Horror Cinema*, and *Kamera*.

ISBN 978-0-399-53303-7

9 780399 533037
51595

$15.95 U.S.
$20.00 CAN

SEXUALITY
www.penguin.com